FREEDOM TO CHOOSE
The Life and Work of Dr Helena Wright
Pioneer of Contraception

FREEDOM TO CHOOSE

BARBARA EVANS

Give women the choice and they will choose . . .
I want to see every individual on earth having
that choice and having it free.

Helena Wright, 1972

THE BODLEY HEAD
LONDON   SYDNEY
TORONTO

For Philip

British Library Cataloguing
in Publication Data
Evans, Barbara Dr
Freedom to choose.
The Life and Work of Dr Helena Wright
Pioneer of Contraception
1. Title
613'94'0924   HQ764.W/
ISBN 0-370-30504-3

© Barbara Evans 1984
Printed in Great Britain for
The Bodley Head Ltd.,
9 Bow Street, London, WC2E 7AL
by Redwood Burn, Trowbridge
set in Linotron Plantin by
Rowland Phototypesetting Ltd
Bury St Edmunds, Suffolk
First published 1984

2257794

CONTENTS

ACKNOWLEDGEMENTS

To Elizabeth Aldwinckle I offer warm thanks for her care and skill in the preparation of the manuscript. I should also like to thank those who have helped me with advice and information, particularly Mary Ainslie, Margaret Allen, the Association of British Adoption and Fostering Agencies, the Apollo Theatre Manager, Dr Harold Wykeham Balme, Professor David Balme, Dame Josephine Barnes, Peter Baylis, the BBC, Ralph Beyer, Freda Bromhead, Princess Birabongse, Daphne Charters, Margaret Cone, Patricia Downie (Faber and Faber), the Family Planning Association, the Fawcett Library (City of London Polytechnic), Charis Frankenburgh, the Garrick Theatre Manager, Lady Houghton, Dr Geraldine Howard, Dr Jean Infield, the International Planned Parenthood Federation, Daphne Jones, Philip Kestelman, Dr Ronald Kleinman, Mira Leslie, Lady Medawar, Naomi Mitchison, Dr Marjorie Myers, Rotha Peers, Sheila Sullivan, Clarence Paget, Dr David Pyke, Diana Rawstron, Cecil Robertson, the Royal Free Hospital Hon. Archivist, the Royal Society of Medicine Librarian, the Society for Chinese Anglo-Understanding, the Victoria and Albert Museum Theatre Museum, the Wellcome Institute for the History of Medicine Contemporary Medical Archives Centre, Jeremy Wright, Dr Margaret Wright, Miranda Wright.

I am particularly appreciative of the time and patience expended by Jill Black of The Bodley Head for whom nothing seemed too much trouble in the production of this book, and whose advice was extremely valuable.

PREFACE

Dr Helena Wright made contraception respectable at a time when the subject was virtually unmentionable in Britain. The early birth control pioneers in the Twenties, among them Marie Stopes, Frida Laski, Dora Russell, Ruth Dalton, Eleanor Rathbone and Mary Stocks, encountered not only public abuse but active medical hostility. When during the Thirties a small group of women founded the Family Planning Association, Helena Wright was the only doctor among them.

For her, contraception was much more than a way of preventing the birth of unwanted babies. It was first a discovery, then a mission and finally the greatest single service which could be offered to families. No longer need mothers be ground down by repeated childbearing, and distracted pregnant girls turned out by affronted parents. Helena Wright believed the service was ideally provided by specially trained women doctors. She conceded that a male doctor was preferable to no doctor, but few men in her opinion were blessed with the sympathy, understanding and gentleness which the new specialty called for. Without the arrogance of Marie Stopes, who alienated doctors nearly as much as she antagonised the Roman Catholic Church, by the mid Thirties Helena had gained acceptance of the principle of contraception from the Anglican bishops. She gradually changed the opinions of the medical hierarchy and made contraception a specialty in its own right.

Contraception gave women the sexual freedom for which Helena Wright campaigned throughout her long life. Having freed countless women from the tormenting fear of pregnancy, she taught them to understand and enjoy their sexuality. Marriage ceased to be 'the price men paid for sex, and sex the price women paid for marriage'. Her views on extramarital sexual activity shocked many people, and aroused criticism which would not be heard today, but she warned that 'The new liberty is not going to make decisions on sexual

7

behaviour any easier than before. Instead the demands on character are harder than they were when behaviour was based on convention and fear.'

I did not meet Dr Wright during her active medical career although I had long known of her in my own professional life as the doyenne of contraception, one of the chief architects of the Family Planning Association and an influential founder of the International Planned Parenthood Federation. Many of my friends and my medical colleagues had been her patients or her pupils or both. She was the great authority of the day to whom 'everybody' went for contraceptive advice.

One day in the late Seventies when I was shopping in our local village bakery in North London I heard talk of the amazing veteran woman doctor, 'must be nearly ninety', who still went all over the world and had just come back from lecturing on birth control in India. I realised that *the* Helena Wright and I were neighbours. I found that she lived alone in an old-fashioned block in St John's Wood. She had christened her flat 'the Bird Cage' when she and her husband, the surgeon H. W. S. Wright, moved there in 1972 from the large family house nearby in which she had brought up her four boys. She furnished the flat with antiques from her father's opulent Paris apartment. She kept her records, dating back even to her schooldays, in four Chinese lacquer cabinets depicting the seasons, each of which had cost ten shillings over fifty years earlier when she and her husband had been missionaries in China.

I usually went to see her on Monday afternoons, which she kept free for me. On other days there would perhaps be visitors from India, China, Europe or North America whom she allowed me to meet. Like her mother, she appeared to have thrown nothing away. She generously made all her documents, letters and manuscripts available to me without restrictions or conditions. She was the biographer's dream. She had technically retired at the age of eighty-five but only from the clinical care of patients. She was still fervently concerned with women, any she had helped, any who still needed help. Leaving me to work on her books and papers, she used to sleep in her chair in the afternoons. Then we would have tea or orange juice – always with clean napkins—and I would record our conversations on her life experiences or her philosophy.

She believed strongly in the paranormal and in life in the Fourth Dimension, and often spoke of the communications she had regularly with her dead husband and others 'on the other side', sometimes prefacing her remarks with the words, 'It's all phoney to you.' Indeed I did find some of her views incongruously eccentric at times, and in sharp contrast with her scientific background. It was impossible to offend her, and if we disagreed she would laugh and change the subject. She believed, as she said, 'Today's cranks are tomorrow's prophets.'

She was always helpful, considerate and understanding. Shortly before her death she wrote to me to explain a point which had arisen in discussion:

My *dear* Barbara,
Our conversation yesterday illuminated for me the extensive mists through which you are conscientiously trying to find a path . . .
                              HRW to author—Bird Cage, 14.5.81
She ended: 'With much sympathy for you—Helena'.

She was invariably cheerful and optimistic, even during the last months of her life when she became easily tired. Her son Adrian told me that he saw his mother seriously distressed only on three occasions: once when his father who had been ill failed to return home after three weeks' absence; again when her great friend Bruce McFarlane died suddenly while they were out together; and lastly at the unexpected death in circumstances to which she had contributed of her son Christopher, when she was distraught.

This book is the story of her life. It is drawn from her own books, letters and papers, and the recollections and writing of her friends, colleagues and critics. I have devoted considerable space to Helena's background and early life because this explains much of her later life and work. I was also given access, with Helena Wright's permission, to a series of helpful tapes she and others had recorded after the death of her distinguished sister, the child psychiatrist Dr Margaret Lowenfeld, when a joint biography of the two sisters was under consideration but did not materialise.

I cannot adequately express my gratitude to Helena's family for all the help they have given me, to her cousin Till Haberfeld and her friend Joan Rettie. I owe especial thanks to Dr Beric Wright who first suggested I should write his mother's biography, thus introducing me to a truly remarkable Victorian with twentieth-century vision.

                                                    FEBRUARY 1983

[I]

In the Beginning

Although she was born in England and lived there all her long life, Dr
Helena Wright did not consider herself English. She was proud to be a
hybrid. Her father Heinz Lowenfeld had spent his youth in the Polish
part of Austria. His forebears were Jewish by race and religion,
although by the end of the nineteenth century many had abandoned
their religion and some had married outside the Jewish faith. Heinz's
father, Emmanuel, belonged to a provincial Prussian family of respected wealthy Jewish landowners, whose estates included property
in Austrian Poland. Emmanuel went to the public grammar school in
Breslau (now Wroclaw) in Silesia, and then to the university where he
studied medicine. He abandoned medicine when his elder brother
died and he then took over the family mining business.

Emmanuel married Rosa Ascher, an unusual Jewish lady, some of
whose characteristics were evident in her granddaughter Helena. She
was an outspoken critical agnostic—though she later became a Roman Catholic—independent and indomitable. She came from an
intellectual Prussian family of artists and writers with a cosmopolitan
background and had lived during part of her childhood in England.
She spoke German, French, Italian and English fluently.

When the Lowenfeld mining business failed after the Crimean
War, bankrupting Emmanuel, Rosa was more than equal to this
unexpected change in their fortunes. She used to visit her husband in
Breslau gaol in her elegant horse-drawn carriage and within five years
with her help they were able to buy back from the Receiver their
Polish estate, with its 2,000 acres of agricultural land, and the 10,000
acres of woodland which had supplied the Lowenfeld iron-ore mines
with timber.

They left Breslau and city life in 1859, the year in which Heinz,
their third son and Helena's father, was born, and moved to this
remote area,Chrzanow, near the Silesian border. There they successfully reclaimed the woodlands, built roads and over forty buildings.

Rosa supervised the renovation and the extensions to the main house and developed the park. Her garden in the English style, unlike the formal French gardens which were popular at the time, had English shrubs and roses. Emmanuel developed an iron-ore industry and built a smelting furnace. He acquired the rights to run a slaughter-house and to distil alcohol, and raised their four sons in comfortable security.

Divided by three separate partitions between Russia, Austria and Prussia, Poland had ceased to exist as an individual state in 1795, and was not to regain her independence until 1918. The Polish community in the 'Three Kingdoms' where the Lowenfelds now lived was either Catholic or Jewish. Neither Protestant Prussia nor Orthodox Russia offered any encouragement to the Polish minority; the Russians were actively hostile to the Poles and only the Austrians were friendly. Rosa, who knew no Polish when they first arrived at Chrzanow, learnt within a year to speak the language. As her sympathy for the suppressed Poles developed, she embraced their cause. In the doomed Polish rebellion of 1863 Rosa, now a fervent Polish patriot, carried messages hidden in her clothing across the Russian frontier twelve kilometres away. She nursed an officer who had taken part in the uprising until he died of his wounds in Chrzanow, and gave other insurgents sanctuary. She became a legend in the village she and Emmanuel had created.

Their eldest boy, Willi, went to the local school until in 1862 Rosa decided to consult her friend and admirer Hugo Gutsche, a philosophy student in Breslau who was about to take his examinations, about Willi's future education. In due course Hugo arrived at Chrzanow, and to the great distress of his own family never returned to them. Some time after his arrival at Chrzanow Rosa's fourth son, Bruno, was born. In his unpublished monograph, *Seventy-six Years of Chrzanow*, Adolf Lowenfeld, the second son, recalls that Bruno had black eyes and was 'different from the rest of us'. 'Pan' (a title of respect) Hugo remained with the Lowenfelds for thirty-six years, first as tutor to the four boys and then as 'Uncle Hugo', a member of the family.

Meanwhile forestry had ceased to be profitable and Emmanuel then put the estate down to agriculture. He rented out some of the fields, closed his distillery and was obliged to mortgage some of the property. He was, however, able to agree with the military authorities to house a squadron of *uhlans*, to erect barracks with special accommodation for the cavalry captain and to improvise stalls for a hundred horses. The garrison of aristocratic officers brought new life and an illusion of prosperity to Chrzanow. Financial problems recurred but Rosa and Emmanuel carried out their fight for existence while their sons lived in happy carefree oblivion of their parents' difficulties. There were balls, skating parties and expeditions.

In September 1880 there arrived at Chrzanow Pan Hugo's niece Elise Bail from Danzig and Alice Evens, a seventeen-year-old girl from London. Alice's parents were friends of Rosa's brother Dr Ascher who worked in the British Museum. Alice had been in poor health and Dr Ascher suggested the trip would do her good. In order to amuse themselves and please their father the young people arranged an impromptu play for Emmanuel's birthday on 1 October, when Heinz would have returned from military service. The only son who did not wear a beard and the most like his father, he would play the part of Emmanuel. Adolf was to play an engineer who had come to supervise the building of the barracks, but had fallen in love with a young English girl he had met on the train (Alice), and Bruno, who spoke Polish best, was to be a servant and make the jokes.

On 29 September Heinz turned up unexpectedly, having cut short his military service by two days. The military authorities treated this as desertion and compulsorily returned him to Dresden the following day. He was kept in Königstein for three months, but Alice was still at Chrzanow when he returned. However, he missed his father's last birthday and Adolf took over the part destined for Heinz.

With Emmanuel's death the following year the dismal financial position of the family lands was revealed. During his last years Emmanuel had had a series of strokes and had been unable to manage the various enterprises. The estate was in debt and in disrepair, and it was clear that if everything was not to be sold the boys would have to earn their livings. Showing remarkable business acumen, Heinz arranged for the sale of part of the property with rights of re-purchase within six years. Adolf went to train as a teacher and Willi as a lawyer in Berlin. Bruno, then nineteen, remained for the time being at Chrzanow.

Leaving Rosa and the faithful Pan Hugo in charge of the remainder of the property, Heinz, now twenty-five, decided to seek his fortune in England. He left with the proverbial five pounds in his pocket, no training and no contacts in England except Alice Evens. She was the daughter of a naval captain, Henry Evens, of whom little is known, except that he was ADC to the Duke of Cambridge, Commander-in-Chief of the British Army. Henry Evens lived with his wife Jane and his five daughters in a large house in the London suburb of Dulwich where there was a lake in the garden. Heinz became a member of the family. His brothers had all tried to seduce Alice at Chrzanow, but she fell in love with Heinz totally and uncritically—Helena described it as an infatuation. In December 1884 they were married and Heinz returned to Chrzanow on his honeymoon with Alice for the first time since his departure.

Alice was shy and inexperienced, small and pale but socially ambitious. Her family was Nonconformist Christian, his was mainly Jewish with a sprinkling of atheists and free-thinkers but included Lutherans and Catholics. Apart from a shared love of horses she and Heinz had little in common. Where she was English, orthodox and conventional, he was Continental, unorthodox and eccentric. He had charm and looks and all he needed was money. Almost immediately he turned out to be a financial genius. Within six years he had redeemed the Chrzanow fortunes, bought from his brothers their shares in the estate, and raised an annuity for his mother. As sole owner he became responsible for all the Chrzanow outgoings.

In England everything he touched turned to gold. He made money by buying and selling at auctions, beginning with Swiss cuckoo clocks and jewellery, but anything would be considered, even on one occasion half a hen-coop. From a modest beginning and by applying the principle 'Buy cheap, sell dear', he moved into property and high finance, taking enormous trouble to make every project profitable.

Early in 1890 Henry Lowenfeld, as he now called himself although he had retained his Austrian nationality, passed an open door in South London. From within came men's voices and, entering uninvited, he found himself at a temperance meeting, where the speaker on the platform was expounding on the evils of alcohol. He heard a member of the audience say, 'Give me a substitute for alcoholic drinks, and I will turn teetotaller at once.' The lecturer had no satisfactory reply, but Henry had. He decided to explore the possibilities of an alternative drink for the working man. In the British Museum Library he read all he needed to know about brewing, and without any previous knowledge acquired enough chemical know-how to formulate an alcohol-free beverage which tasted like beer.

He then bought a six-acre field by the river at Fulham and, at a cost of nearly £50,000, built a model brewery on half the land, using the remaining three acres for storage, packing sheds and stabling. By 1892 the brewery was turning out 75,000 pints a day of a fermented drink which Henry christened 'Kop's Ale'. It was made from Kentish hops and was, so ran the advertisements, 'entirely free from the taint of alcohol'. It was distributed throughout London by Lowenfeld drays, which bore the name in large letters. Handbills publicised Kop's Ale and Stout, 'the ideal drink for cyclists. Available wholesale only from Kop's Brewery, Wandsworth Bridge, Fulham.' For the public it was 'to be obtained at all hostelries, cyclist resorts and headquarters, and of all grocers, wine merchants etc. in the United Kingdom'.

Mr Lowenfeld was his own public relations officer. On 23 November 1891, the year in which his brewery was completed, he delivered a lecture on 'Drink and Drunkenness' at the St James's Hall, Piccadilly, to the Balloon Society of Great Britain, a popular scientific, literary and art society of the day. The *Daily Mirror*, reporting this event, quoted Mr Henry Lowenfeld as saying that England was spending '£66 million a year on wines and spirits, £85½ million on beer, and consumed 17 gallons of beer against each one gallon of wines and spirits, or three times as much alcohol in the shape of beer compared with all other alcoholic drinks. The beer consumption in England was a quarter larger than in Germany, three times as large as in Austria, five times as large as in France and 26 times that of Russia.' Moreover, Mr Lowenfeld had had it from that well-known physician Sir Andrew Clarke that 'seven out of every ten cases in his hospital were caused by alcoholic drink'.

Once Kop's Ale was on the market Henry Lowenfeld contrived to interest the press in his product. On 28 April 1892 *Christian World* reported favourably on the brewery where its columnist 'Rambler' had been able to meet Mr Lowenfeld, 'a short, dark, springy gentleman of 40 to 45 with a slight German accent'. More importantly the medical press was well disposed. On 9 April 1892 a writer in *Family Doctor* recalled that the previous autumn he had had the pleasure of paying a visit of inspection to 'the huge establishment where this renowned non-alcoholic beverage (Kop's Ale) is brewed', and had left with the

. . . homely but enthusiastic eulogium passed by a perspiring and thirsty stone mason ringing in his ears, 'There's not a headache in a hogshead, and to work on in summer it beats all your ale and porter hollow.'

The product was investigated by the *Lancet* Special Analytical Commission on Mineral Waters, Temperance Beverages, etc., which found the preparation was based on sound scientific principles. In July 1892 the *Lancet* reported:

> Kop's Ale has a right to the title of a non-intoxicating beverage as an excellent substitute for ordinary ale, which it resembles in taste, colour and composition . . . The public and especially the teetotal public may evidently drink Kop's Ale with confidence. It contains nothing that is injurious, but is on the contrary, a salutary and palatable beverage possessing distinct tonic and stimulating properties by virtue of the choice ingredients which form the basis of its preparation.

Apart from hops the four main ingredients in Kop's Ale were horehound, 'one of the most beneficial of bitter herbs', ginger, dandelion root and cane sugar for the yeast fermentation. The commissioner who had visited the brewery found

> . . . everything was laid open to his inspection and not a single operation in the whole brewery was allowed to escape his notice, albeit there were many steps in the process of a secret nature.

Kop's Ale could hardly fail to prosper, and older members of the population still remember it with satisfaction. Eventually Henry lost interest, and moved on to other projects. He sold out to the White brothers of ginger-beer fame. When they gathered to sign the transfer, Henry Lowenfeld discovered that the goodwill had not been included in the contract note, 'Never mind,' said Henry, 'we'll make it £1,000 for every letter in the name.' 'Thank goodness it's a short one,' said the White brothers, as they agreed on another £4,000 for the goodwill of Kop's.

That was the end of Kop's Ale as far as Henry Lowenfeld was concerned. I have described the development of the project in some detail to illustrate his methods, his ability and versatility. But it was only one of numerous successful enterprises conceived by his fertile mind. He was already interested in real estate and in the previous years had been developing a finance company, the Universal Stock Exchange Ltd., later the Investment Registry Ltd. In this he dealt directly with the public in stocks and shares as a jobber, doing away with commissions over four per cent, which saved money for the small investors, those below the £10,000 limit and relatively inexperienced in the theory and practice of investment. He operated from Waterloo Place, in London, where the business occupied the whole of a large house.

In 1893 the *Daily Chronicle* announced that the *Pall Mall Gazette* had changed hands, having been purchased by Mr T. Dove Keighley, formerly acting manager of the Avenue Theatre (now the Playhouse). It was rumoured that he was acting for Mr Henry Lowenfeld, and this was indeed the case; the Keighleys were friends of the Lowenfelds. The reason Henry used a third party is not clear, but according to Helena there had been arguments between Henry and the editor.

In the same year, 1893, Henry Lowenfeld acquired the lease of the Prince of Wales Theatre which he managed until 1898. Here he was the first person to erect advertising posters on the outside walls of a London theatre. He also had a financial interest in the Lyric Theatre and eventually owned his own theatre, the Apollo, which he built in 1900. Early that year he had noticed the irregularly-shaped vacant site in Shaftesbury Avenue at the corner of Rupert Street, next to the Lyric Theatre, seen its possibilities and bought the freehold. Shaftesbury Avenue had been opened in 1887, the year of Helena's birth, and was to become the main artery of theatreland, running from the newly constructed Piccadilly Circus to New Oxford Street. The Shaftesbury was the first and the Lyric the second theatre to be built in this new road. The Palace Theatre was the third, then came Henry's Apollo.

The theatre opened on 21 February 1901 with a musical, appropriately entitled *The Belle of Bohemia*. Henry had spent the year in which the theatre was being built learning the ropes, including casting and direction from his friend and associate, George Edwardes, the manager of Daly's Theatre. As was his habit, Henry had taken enormous trouble over every detail. The building is entirely without pillars, except on the top floor in the room he used as his office. The façade is in the French renaissance style and Henry had himself designed the orchestra pit as an adaptation of Wagner's construction at Bayreuth, intended to produce the right sound relationships of the various instruments.

When the gypsies on the Polish Chrzanow estate learnt of the enterprise in which young Mr Lowenfeld was engaged in London, their chief presented him with a silver ornament on a chain, to bring him luck. This was their emblem, and depicts a flying serpent between two lions rampant, reproduced on the jacket of this book. Henry immediately conceived the motif as embodying his initials, the front paws of the lions forming the cross bar of the H and their bodies the uprights, with the serpent's tail the L, and this became his logo, or personal crest.

The ornament was framed and hung in the foyer of the Apollo, and its design was incorporated throughout the fabric of the theatre, on the curtain, the carpeting, the back of every seat and on the external wall, where it can still be seen by the main door. It was used in the programmes and even appeared on the matchboxes distributed on the opening night. This performance was widely publicised, and the *Sketch* on 27 February 1901, in the year of Queen Victoria's death, noted that:

> Of course the event of the past week was the opening of the new playhouse, at present called the 'Apollo Theatre', for it is believed that Mr Lowenfeld may change the name to one associated with that of the new King.

Henry had caused a furore by restricting admission on the first night to an invited audience consisting of his friends, the critics, managers and staff of other theatres, and potential patrons. The *Sketch* protested that:

> . . . critics cannot or should not make up their minds without the assistance of the public at a first night performance . . . There was a prodigious crowd at the invitation performance . . . and most people seemed delighted by the gorgeous decoration of the house. Some critics pretended that there was less taste than gold used in the treatment.

Henry lost interest in the Apollo in 1904 but he put a manager into the theatre until 1920, when he sold it. Being a superstitious man he attributed all his theatrical success to the gypsy's gift, which his grandson Michael Wright has to this day. Even more, perhaps, than the gypsy's gift Henry valued his 'lucky' threepenny bit, which he left in his will to his eldest grandson, Beric Wright. He had acquired it when he stopped to buy a paper soon after his arrival in England and had been given this coin by mistake in his change. As soon as she saw she had given it to Henry the newspaper girl asked for it back, as she declared it was her lucky coin. On it Henry saw the letter H on one side and refused to oblige the girl. Until then things had not been going well, but the following day he found to his surprise 'conciliation where he had looked for stern enactment, confidence for distrust and kindness for suspicion'. Thereafter he kept the lucky piece in his string purse together with six other threepenny bits which he termed the 'courtiers of the King'.

Helena Rosa Lowenfeld was born in Tulse Hill Road, in Brixton, in 1887 while Henry was still relatively poor, but by the time his second daughter Margaret was born in 1890 he was on the way to becoming a small tycoon, and had prospered sufficiently to move to a more substantial house. One afternoon he hired a pony carriage, collected Alice and drove over the river to Knightsbridge. They drew up outside a large double-fronted five-storeyed house in Lowndes Square. 'This is where we are going to live,' said Henry. The house had once been occupied by the American Minister in London, a Mr Phelps, but because it was infested the owner had had difficulty in selling the lease. 'What are a few fleas?' asked Henry, and got the house cheaply.

[2]

London Childhood

Helena and Margaret Lowenfeld grew up in the large house in Lowndes Square in conditions of increasingly extravagant luxury. Henry, giving them the barest directions, employed three well-known firms to furnish the principal rooms. Helena remembered that the 'Japanese' room had handsome embroidered pelmets. The main drawing-room was furnished by Maples with an Aubusson carpet on which stood original Louis x v tapestry chairs and a grand piano. The ballroom contained only gold spindly chairs. Of the three guest rooms Helena thought the 'Italian' one dark and gloomy. The nurseries were on the fourth floor and the indoor servants, cook, kitchenmaid, head housemaid and under housemaid, slept on the fifth floor. The outdoor servants and the footmen lived in the mews at the back with the horses.

The menservants wore the Lowenfeld blue livery with silver buttons stamped with the initials H L, except Kelly, the Irish butler, who wore tails. He slept in the basement on a folding bed which was relegated to a cupboard by day. Margaret, always known in the family as 'Madge', noted in her diary when she was ten that a domestic pet, 'Chow Chow', got shut in Kelly's bed and suffocated. Kelly was known by his real surname and so was Bickmore, the coachman, but the other servants changed so frequently that the grooms were always called 'William' and the footmen 'Henry'. Kelly's identical twin brother was a butler in neighbouring Belgrave Square. The twins would sometimes change places without their respective employers being aware which twin was serving them, and neither ever said.

Life in Lowndes Square revolved around Henry Lowenfeld. He was the dominating influence in the running of the establishment. Alice was subservient and devoted. She scrupulously pasted into her cuttings-book, which survived her, all press and other notices of his public activities, whether relating to Kop's Ale or the world of the theatre. He continued to make money and to enjoy himself. Every night he returned an hour before dinner to an orderly and well-run establishment to which Alice, with six indoor and three outdoor servants, herself totally inexperienced in the domestic arts, had not contributed more than the five minutes required for the morning consultation with the Swedish cook. Though the girls thought her a crosspatch Henry appreciated the cook's art and once at the end of dinner sent Kelly to his study to fetch a leather case from his bureau drawer and asked him to convey it to Cook with his compliments and to say he hoped she would like the brooch inside. Henry could also be awkward—on one occasion which Helena recalled he ordered Kelly to inform all his wife's dinner guests as they arrived that the party was cancelled. He was given to occasional rages which caused Margaret to dissolve into tears. Not so Helena. She was determined that her father, to his annoyance, should not make her cry.

Alice was pleased to be the wife of a successful and important public figure. She was presented at Court in 1897, the year of Queen Victoria's Jubilee and occupied herself at Lowndes Square with fashionable London life, supporting Tory organisations such as the Primrose League and other ladylike activities. Much of her energy went into the role of elegant hostess. Margaret noted in her diary when she was nine: 'She entertained a great deal, giving musical at homes at which I handed round ices.' Alice's Thursday afternoons became part of the London scene, and were noticed in the press. Thus *Kensington Society*, 11 May 1893:

Mrs Henry Lowenfeld gave a delightful At Home last Thursday afternoon at her beautiful house at 31 Lowndes Square. Music was the attraction, and it was of the best possible to procure. The lovely rooms were filled during the afternoon by a smart set of guests who much enjoyed the singing of Madame Belle Cole and Mrs Wallace Brownlow, and the violin solo of Mr René Payne, as well as the piano playing of Senor Albeniz. Mrs Lowenfeld was an indefatigable hostess and the afternoon proved a great success. There was some excellent music as indeed there always is, Mrs Lowenfeld's taste being well known. Charles Copland gave an excellent rendering of *The Berceuse* and *Love me if I live* and Miss Elsie Lincoln sang with great artistic powers *Spring Time* and *Printemps Nouveau*. Senor Albeniz, the talented author of *The Magic Ring*, gave a brilliant piano solo and Miss Bardia and Madame Square also assisted. The hostess looked well in the palest blue crepe de chine with insertions of green velvet, the yoke and trimmings of pale green silk and lace.

On another occasion—19 April 1894—Alice was described as wearing 'A smart gown of sky-blue cashmere with reveres of black moiré'.

Alice kept her own records, like any good hostess, of the food served to her guests. This is the menu at her At Home on 15 June 1893:

Clear Soup

Salmon Fillets.   Briton Sauce
Garnished Crayfish   Lobster Mayonnaise

Raised Chicken Pie   Veal and Ham Pie
Pigeon Pie   Pressed Beef   Ham
Stuffed Quails   Pigeons à la Provençale   Cutlets à la Calgège
Roast Fowls   Tongue   Foie Gras in Aspic

Chartreuse Gâteau à la Mocha
Nougat Pudding   Baba Cake
Pineapple Cream Tartlets
Meringues   Chocolate Eclairs   Jellies

This elaborate assortment seems to have been fairly typical. On 9 February 1893 three courses were served for supper, exclusive of 'Chicken and Ham, Caviare, Anchovies and Foie Gras sandwiches, with Forcemeat Rolls and Dessert'.

By the end of the century Alice had become interested in spiritualism, and Margaret's diary in 1900 refers to the fact that it took up more and more of her mother's time: 'There always seemed to be seances going on in the house.'

At the time of their marriage Henry Lowenfeld had warned Alice that fidelity was not to be included in the contract. He proposed to keep mistresses in the Continental fashion but they would not impinge on family life, and his wife and mistresses would never meet. No affair would last longer than a year because after a year an affair would become a relationship, and this was something he did not wish to develop. Alice presumably agreed to this arrangement to which Henry kept faithfully for sixteen years. The girls were only to learn later of it from Alice, but as time passed they began to see a pattern developing in their parents' relationship which, although it puzzled them, was never openly discussed in the early stages, although from Helena's subsequent correspondence it is clear that she at least was aware of developing discord between her parents. However, Alice appeared ignorant of Henry's liaisons with women who were mainly actresses associated with his theatrical interests. With the women involved he was open and straightforward; the position was established from the start that it would be held for only a year. No false expectations were to be raised, no cause for jealousy need arise. During her year in office Henry would provide for the lady's needs in comfortable, luxurious accommodation on the understanding that she would remain available solely for him at any time of the day or night. In after years, when Helena met a number of his women friends, each told her that their year with Henry was 'the best in their lives'.

Henry had a somewhat similar arrangement with the Spanish composer and pianist Ysidor Albeniz, a pupil of Liszt, who in 1891 had obtained permission from the Queen of Spain—he was the official court pianist—to come to England. Henry Lowenfeld heard him play at a concert in London and there and then entered into an agreement whereby for a handsome retainer Albeniz would make himself available day or night, to play at Lowndes Square to Henry whenever the fancy took him to hear some music. Helena used to listen to Albeniz playing to her father on the upright piano in the morning room, and so became conditioned at an early age to a love of music, one of the great pleasures of her adult life. The arrangement suited Albeniz perfectly because, with a family to support, he could spend his spare time composing instead of performing in public. He wrote the music for the comic opera *The Magic Opal* which opened at the Lyric Theatre in 1893 and, renamed *The Magic Ring*, transferred to the Prince of Wales, now leased by Henry Lowenfeld and under his management.

Meanwhile the two girls saw little of their mother, who paid increasingly less and less attention to them. They were relegated to the care of Nurse Minter. They lunched with their mother in the dining-room and were sent down from the nurseries to the morning room to see her for half an hour at four o'clock if she was not entertaining her friends or holding one of her 'Thursdays'.

It was Nurse Minter's boast that her charges were the best-dressed children in the Park. There, dressed by Debenhams, Woollands or Harvey Nichols, they were instructed to walk in front of her while she conversed with other nurses similarly employed. Some mornings

Helena and Margaret would ride in Rotten Row with their father, who as often as not would meet some of his business friends and would make the girls ride behind him. At Albert Gate he would send them back down Knightsbridge, unescorted, to Lowndes Square while he cantered off. Buses could be a hazard and there was a right-hand turn into the Square to manoeuvre. Helena grew up hating Hyde Park, horses and dressing up, and these dislikes lasted all her life.

There is little doubt, however, that both girls were at that time extremely fond of their father. Thus Margaret, writing at the age of six from Poland:

> My darling Papa
> I am very sorry that I have not written before but I will write a nice long letter for your birthday which I hope will be happy my own Darling Papa . . . Try to guess what we are making for your present I am sure you will say it is very useful it is for your dressing table. My first tooth has come out I pulled it out all by myself. Miss Constant said I was very brave . . . Please to answer as quickly as possible these letters. Good bye my darling Papa
> With much love and kisses from
> Your own
> Baby
>
> ML to HL—Chrzanow, August 1896

The page ends with three rows of crosses and the numerals 140, in case the financial wizard could not count. Two years later, on 18 September 1898, Margaret, writing from the Gartenhaus to 'Darling Papa' was still ending her letter 'Love from your loving little daughter Baby'.

Eight years old and still 'Baby'? The significance is not far to seek. She was an unhappy child, frequently ailing and left alone for hours or days in bed in Lowndes Square in the care of servants. The only one she liked was Kelly whom she adored, but he was hardly likely to have been able to spend much time in the night nursery. She later recalled having 'night terrors and screaming fits', and she was given to thumb-sucking which was 'very difficult to break'. In later letters she revealed that her mother never showed her any warmth or affection; Margaret once heard her say with exasperation, 'Is that child ill *again*?' Helena has confirmed this apparent indifference on her mother's part towards her children. Many years later, when she had children of her own she wrote to her mother from China, explaining that she did not propose to bring them up on the pattern of her own childhood:

> My darling Mother
> . . .I can't remember anything before Lowndes Square; there to me you were merely a shadow, a shadow with three characteristics; you were always 'busy' and you were always either ill or worried. I never remember you happy at all. Madge and I saw you as we went out for our detested morning walk, when you were invariably buried in writing at your desk, at lunch, and sometimes after tea in the morning room. I don't remember that you once spent time actually playing with us in the nursery. If you did it wasn't often enough to make any impression. I mean when we were small—or indeed at any time.
>
> Nurse Minter was our chief companion. I realised *very* early that she was a servant and not our equal. I knew she was stupid and didn't attempt to get any companionship out of her . . . Why didn't you get to know your children a little? . . . But you were chasing the social will o' the wisp and hadn't the time . . .
>
> From about the age of seven to nine the only thing I can remember you doing with me was making me come for drives in the Park in the Season. How anyone could imagine that would interest a lively healthy child I don't know; anyway it didn't me. I can still feel the sense of deadly boredom as we went slowly backwards and forwards among all the other people in *their* stupid carriages.
>
> HRW to AQ[1]—Peking, 7.6.22

Her own maternal technique differed sharply from that of her mother, as she indicated in a subsequent letter:

> I take good care to be the centre of my children's lives and am succeeding . . . I watch everything, but make them feel as free as possible . . . I expect to go along with them, loving but never criticising all their friends, hearing all their interests, but do not

---

[1] Alice Lowenfeld remarried in April 1907, becoming Mrs Frank Quicke. Letters written to her before that date are noted A L, those afterwards A Q.

expect them to be interested in my affairs. I mean to keep my own vivid individual life and interests apart and independent of them, so that when my day is over and they go (which of course they will) I will still have a full and useful life to pursue . . . I expect them to have new radical views, be more progressive than we are, and I don't care tuppence if they agree with my views or not.

HRW to AQ—Tsinan, 12.12.26

Helena was the more resilient of the sisters. She was also the leader. It was Helena who, at the age of six, announced out of the blue one day at lunch before she even knew the meaning of the word that she was going to be a doctor when she grew up. Predictably Margaret followed suit in due course, to the enormous disgust of their father who wished them to be conventional English girls who would eventually marry bankers. 'What has fate done to give me two intelligent daughters?' he is alleged to have exclaimed. Both made distinguished careers, Helena in the field of contraception and sexual medicine, and Margaret as a renowned child psychiatrist. Margaret had a highly original mind and was to found the Institute of Child Psychology in London. She was an innovator of play therapy for normal but disturbed children, and the diagnostic tests she devised as a means of understanding children's problems were used and adapted, after a visit to the ICP, by that distinguished anthropologist Margaret Mead in her work with primitive peoples.

In spite of her many later achievements, life posed a series of problems for Margaret Lowenfeld. She had great difficulty in carrying out her ingenious ideas. She could not express them, and she was not, like Melanie Klein, a good collaborator. While Helena, who did almost no scientific research, left six books to posterity, some of Margaret's work was only published after her death by her close companion and Danish colleague at the Institute, Ville Andersen. By contrast, everything went Helena's way. She was successful and efficient, practical and businesslike and, unlike Margaret, had a stable income. Ville Andersen believed that Margaret's 'failure to prepare for her retirement or to regard money as a necessity was to some extent due to her disgust for her father's wealth, which had made her childhood so lonely and miserable'. Helena never knew poverty, and found her father's money handy in her youth, although she has said, 'We had the misfortune to be very rich and that made our lives as children very dull.' Nevertheless, money gave her security and self-assurance in the early days of her career. But at the end of an immensely successful life she left just over £8,000 in stocks and shares and money, and no property.

Margaret always felt she had to compete with her gifted and successful elder sister to whom everything came so easily while she herself found everything difficult. According to their cousin Gunther Lowenfeld, who loved both sisters and was grateful to them for helping him and his family in England when they left Germany to avoid Nazi persecution in 1938: 'Madge always felt less successful than Helena and that doomed her whole youth . . . While Madge was always struggling . . . Helena was satisfied with herself, her friends, her life, everything.' Even at the end of Margaret's life, while her health was failing, Helena, then eighty-five, was lecturing all over India.

In due course both girls went to kindergarten, Helena first, in the mornings, to the Froebel Educational Institution in Talgarth Road in West Kensington, said to be the first Froebel school in England. She remembered this as an enjoyable time and thought the school well run. She was 'very backward' at reading but got splendid reports in arithmetic and grammar, and her conduct was 'always satisfactory'. The headmistress, Esther Laurence, wrote of her: 'Is a bright interesting girl, who thinks well. I am very sorry she is leaving the school. Winter Term 1895—absent 14 times—late 11.'

Her next school in Queen's Gate appears to have made little impact, apart from one lasting effect. A little boy, exactly Helena's age, Oliver Hill, also went to the same school. He was the youngest of seven children who lived opposite and Helena thought his mother neglected him, preferring his older sisters. Perhaps with some fellow-feeling and to make up for his loneliness at home, Helena took him under her wing and made him feel valued at Lowndes Square. He was often sulky and rude, and he would sometimes refuse to go to school, but Helena could usually persuade him to do so. When describing their relationship she said later: 'As a child he was the only male who mattered to me at all, apart from my father, but he mattered in a kind of protective way which persisted.'

Oliver Hill became a distinguished architect and remained one of her lifelong friends, sharing with Helena holidays and houses until his marriage at the age of sixty-two to a woman twenty-five years his junior—the 'best offer I ever had', Helena said he told her. From the earliest days of their relationship Helena called him 'Tom', the first recorded instance of her habit of re-christening people, just as she later insisted that her own husband Henry Wright was to be called 'Peter'.

The two little Lowenfeld girls also had a series of governesses, at least five in as many years, German, French, Austrian, Polish, as well as English. There was a Miss Constant (1895), Miss Bittner (1896) who gave them Polish lessons, Miss Crampton (1897) and Miss Pithy (1898). Nurse Minter was still around to see to their clothes, but the governesses would take the girls skating, to Mrs Wordsworth's dancing class or Macpherson's gym. Unless they approved of them Helena and Margaret collaborated in organising the departure of the wretched woman at their mercy. Helena was the motivating force once the decision had been taken to get rid of each one, until in 1898 Nurse Minter disappeared from the scene and Miss Ada Smith, re-christened in the Lowenfeld manner 'Smuttles', arrived. 'Smuttles' remained for many years, and became a loyal friend in the troubled years which were to follow when she became 'The Smut'. Meanwhile Polish language lessons were continued by a Miss Drojecka (1899) who looked after Margaret after school hours when she went on to the Church of England High School in Graham Street at the age of eight.

Both girls retained an abiding interest in Poland. Throughout their childhood they returned at frequent intervals with their parents to their father's by now large family estate, where they shared long summer holidays with three Polish and eight German cousins who spoke no English. These close persisting ties were later to save the Lowenfeld Jews from the gas chambers. 'We collected them,' Helena said. 'They came to us for as long as it was necessary—for months or years.' Some had left before the advent of the Nazis. Among them Margaretta, Willi's daughter and Helena's first cousin, was the only victim. She had married a Gentile and, believing herself thus to be free from the risk of Nazi persecution, returned to Berlin. There she was betrayed and sent to Auschwitz, where no trace of her was found at the liberation. It was thought that she died of starvation.

[3]

School Days

When she was eleven Helena was sent as a weekly boarder to Miss Glatz's school, the Princess Helena College and High School for Girls at Ealing, where she was intensely miserable. Her mother would take her there on Monday mornings and fetch her on Fridays, 'days of pure gold'. 'How poisonously I loathed that unspeakable Miss Glatz, and everything to do with her disgusting little house,' she wrote later to her mother.

> . . . There aren't enough violent words in the language to describe [it]. I learned nothing during that time, my energies were too fully taken up with active misery. The only thing I lived for were Friday afternoons, and then for the first time you, as you, had a really definite value; you represented escape from the horrors of the week. Do you remember my beseeching you not to send me back? Ugh—don't let's talk about that beastly time, even now it makes me shudder.
>
> HRW to AQ—Peking, 7.6.22

Until Helena went to Miss Glatz's school she had no idea how other children lived, and was amazed to find they had different standards in their homes. 'No butlers?' she is alleged to have asked. 'Do they have soap in their houses?' She had never before eaten ordinary food and found school meals unpleasant, tasteless and dull. The pattern emerged of an extrovert child who could not conform. She was unaccustomed to rules and obeyed only those which seemed to her reasonable. Thus she would go to bed and get up in the morning when it suited her, not at the appointed hours. Punishment merely amused her, and she had no sense of guilt at disobeying rules. She had no trace of the herd instinct either, and preferred to sit at the back of the classroom during lessons. When asked if she could see the blackboard, she replied that she couldn't see it in the front row either, 'That's why I'm sitting here.' It transpired that she was short-sighted and needed glasses, which were duly prescribed, but not before she had been sent to a Christian Scientist healer who finally told her mother he was afraid her daughter's mind was 'resistant to truth'.

She got up and left one class at Ealing, taking with her another girl, Flossie, saying to her, 'We can't stand any more of this.' When sent to the headmistress she explained that the teacher was a bad one and it was a waste of time sitting through her lessons. The same teacher had disappeared by the next term, so maybe Helena's diagnosis was correct. But she was not considered a good influence and was not allowed to sleep in a dormitory with other girls. She was put alone in a room on the top floor, 'where the harm I could do was strictly limited'.

As Helena became progressively at cross-purposes with her teachers her school reports deteriorated correspondingly and showed no understanding of the child's character, but much of the obtuseness of the staff. No one commented on the fact that she was a year younger than the average age of the girls in her form, and was consistently good at History, Euclid and Literature, although overall nearer the bottom than the top half of the class. No one seems to have realised that she worked hard for the school charities and was kind and generous. She once deliberately lost a singles match in the tennis tournament: 'I let myself be beaten by a small kid. I gave her the game because it made her happy, therefore it's not so bad as being properly beaten. Now tata darling.' (HRW to AL—21.8.01)

She wrote to her mother, who kept all her letters, two or three times a week, always affectionately.

> My own little darling,
>   The curate from St Peter's is coming next Saturday to give us some lectures on early Church History, interesting!!! Happily they will be in the dark so we can dose [sic].
>   Miss Williamson has given me to do this afternoon, instead of reading, to answer some questions on 'Stories and Teaching on the Litany'. *What* a lot of good it'll do me! How *little* people understand me.
>
>   HRW to AL—3.2.01

> . . . Don't you think it is funny how children quarrel and think it is going to be kept up for years and the next day it is quite all right again? I am making new friends and I think more girls like me than they used to . . . Since the last bust-up I have been

better altogether. Anyhow I feel much *gooder* since I have heard of 'Science'.

H R W to A L—7.2.01

Her letters to Alice usually included requests for articles of clothing to replace those she had left at home or worn out. 'Charlotte' frequently failed to send the right things. 'I've had to wear one pair of combinations for three weeks,' Helena wrote plaintively on one occasion. She had to ask her mother twice for a black skirt for Queen Victoria's funeral.

> My own little darling,
>
> Nearly *all* the girls are in mourning, except one or two. I think I ought to have something black don't you? A black skirt would do if you can't get anything else . . . Now darling Goodbye. With *very very* best love.
>
> P S. I should very much like to see the Queen's funeral.

H R W to A L—27.1.01

Her wish was granted and a room duly taken on the route. She was delighted, but still concerned about her clothes.

> Have you got me a black skirt? if not I shall have to wear one of yours tucked in round the waist and I daresay I can get into one of your black blouses.
>
> Please send the carriage at 3.30. So I shall be home in time for tea. How large is the room? I hope we shall be able to see well, and Oh! I shan't have to *howl all* the time shall I? If so it is a matter of impossibility. I haven't such a store of tears in my body.
>
> Shall we have to get there at about eight? For pity's sake let's have some provisions with us. I shall starve.
>
> I am longing to get home out of the reach of mistresses everlastingly running round after us . . . I am going to come in my brown dress and black coat and hat.
>
> With *best* love darling . . .
>
> P S. How old shall I be when I am presented to the King!!!

H R W to A L—31.1.01

She was perennially broke. At the school bazaar in June 1901 she had spent 2d. on sweets, 3d. on having her hand read by a palmist, 'an utter fraud, she told me a lot of rot', and 3/- on a mat for her mother as a present. She then asked her mother, typically, for a book on palmistry. Helena was often forced to borrow money for stamps as Alice appears to have ignored many repeated requests. 'Don't put them all *outside* the envelope,' Helena once enjoined her mother.

But her major preoccupation was usually her father, and in nearly all her letters she either asked or commented about him and his business. There must have been one particular problem to which Alice had made veiled reference. Thus Helena in March 1901: 'Has the theatre been getting Papa any profits yet?' And a week later when she had heard that the expenses were not covered she suggested giving up violin lessons to save £3 a term, 'but, I don't think I had better give up piano because that will be necessary if I ever want to be any good.' She thought they should 'sell some of the horses and carriages and would then need only one stable at Lowndes Square'. She sent her love to Papa and asked Alice to tell him to cheer up.

In April she wrote; 'I'm sorry about the business, but if it has to come it has and I wish it would make haste about it and not leave us in suspense.' As no one relieved her anxiety she wrote again:

> Are we all bankrupt yet? Tell me what is happening. I have got a few broaches [*sic*] that would fetch about £15 towards the £70,000!!!
>
> HRW to AL—28.4.01

Evidently this was poorly received, and she then explained that she had written 'in sober earnest' and 'wasn't making fun of anything'. She was glad they wouldn't have the bailiffs in. In May she asked again:

> What on earth is that wonderful case of Papa's about . . . What there is such a fuss made over? The girls here very seldom get hold of the papers. If they do it is generally only little village journals. I hope this business is nothing to be ashamed of, as some of papa's actions are at times rather—
>
> HRW to AL—19.5.01

By August she was arranging for ten girls and two members of the staff to go to the theatre, which by then was doing well whatever may have been the outcome of 'the case'. She wrote:

> My own little Darling,
>   I have told the girls and they are nearly off their heads. It *must*

come off. Have you written to Miss Williamson yet? Oh *do* and tell her she *must let* us come. Coax or kiss her or do what you like . . . She has said I may come on Thursday, so that is one load off my mind. Hurrah. How ripping it will be.

HRW to AL—undated.

Besides Flossie, the child of a German baroness, Helena's other friend at the Princess Helena College was another girl like herself of Continental extraction, Ina Kellner. Helena missed Albeniz, but Ina, older and in the sixth form as well as being head girl, was artistic and musical. It comforted Helena who loved music to listen to Ina practising the piano. As for games, she only liked lacrosse; the idea of throwing something up in the air was preferable to chasing a small ball along the ground at hockey. To Helena, lacrosse was a means of self-expression, and she was good enough to play in the first eleven.

Then there was acting, at which she was also good. It was decided that Helena should be the fool Touchstone in the school performance of *As You Like It*. As she said, 'It suited me exactly,' a fair comment as she declaimed: 'I use my folly as a stalking horse for my wit.' Helena was anxious the performance should be a success. It was to be in aid of the Gymnasium Fund and reserved seats were 2/9d. She urged Alice to come and support the Fund of which the proceeds from *As You Like It* were to be the nucleus. 'We have to get as much as we possibly can. You and Papa will help, won't you? We *must* have the Gym.' Alice obliged by taking nine reserved seats, but sadly no further record remains as to how her daughter performed on the night or if she managed, as she hoped, to avoid—a fear expressed many times —'making a fool of myself. I do hope I shan't.'

Even when there was talk of business failure and incipient financial ruin it was always assumed that there would of course be the usual holidays. Relatives and friends came to stay at Lowndes Square at Christmas, where the function was celebrated in the Continental tradition. Festivities began on Christmas Eve, when the main drawing-room was rearranged to give the impression of an exhibition room. The tree, from floor to ceiling, held pride of place in the centre with candles which Kelly lit while the family were having tea and cake in the morning room. The furniture in the drawing-room had been moved, and all round were little tables, one for each person, each covered with a white cloth on which stood a vase of flowers, a basket of fruit and a box of sweets. The presents were laid out on the tables, not on the tree. After tea everyone came upstairs to stand in admiration round the tree—but not to sing, that was a German custom—before moving each to his or her table.

In due course the children went up to bed and the grown-ups settled down to Polish Christmas dinner, which became an institution. In her own home Helena later regularly provided approximately the same menu. They began with lobster soup, followed by a large fish, carp or pike or whatever was available. Fish was considered a great delicacy in the Lowenfelds' part of Poland, an area far from the sea at Gdansk. At Lowndes Square, as in Poland, it was decorated with green capers and accompanied by a special sauce intended to augment the flavour of the somewhat tasteless fish. Then came Polish Christmas pudding and this too Helena learnt to make herself and to serve regularly at Christmas in her own home. It consisted of warmed sweetened milk poured on to slices of white bread, layered with ground almonds and vanilla sugar, topped with poppy seeds. This concoction was eaten cold. On Christmas Day itself the family reverted to typical English Christmas habits with turkey, chestnuts, English plum pudding and brandy sauce for dinner.

Alternate summers were spent either in Poland or on the Isle of Wight. Here Henry had acquired three houses and a public house, and in 1897 he added to his real estate investment the Ocean Hotel at Sandown which he bought to rebuild. Not to be outdone, Alice bought a small villa called Bay View, which Helena thought was a horrid little house. There was not much for Alice to do so she then bought a 'four-in-hand'. With Bickmore, the Lowndes Square coachman, beside her, she amused herself driving about the island. Helena had to go along as well, and was intensely bored by the exercise, but entertained herself by blowing the (mouth) horn from the rear seat, when it was necessary to warn the islanders of their approach. Henry then got himself a similar four-in-hand, but for a different reason. He intended to compete for the record of the fastest time in which to complete the island circuit. To do this he had to discover the existing record, only to find that he could not beat this with his four horses, so he brought over another sixteen and set up four staging posts. At each staging post four horses were changed, and this enabled him to achieve another ambition.

Poland remained his great love, and as far as Henry's children were concerned holidays elsewhere could not compare with summers spent at Chrzanow with his brothers' children. Helena's earliest memory dated from the age of three, looking out on to a snow-covered avenue from her grandmother's old stone house, where the walls and window sills were a metre thick. After Rosa's death in 1898 Adolf returned from Berlin with his family to manage the Chrzanow estate and look after Uncle Hugo until he died. Helena was the eldest of the Lowenfeld cousins, by all accounts a wild bunch, none of whom would even try to speak English with the two 'foreigners', which meant that from an early age Margaret and Helena learnt to speak Polish and to understand German.

Their journey from England was made in the greatest comfort, by the morning train from Victoria in first-class reserved compartments, one for the children and their nurse in which they could play and one for the grown-ups. They then took the Ostend or Calais boat according to the proposed itinerary. Again in first-class reserved carriages they went either via Berlin or Vienna and the other way round on the return journey, sleeping in each city in the Bristol Hotel in their usual reserved suites. Chrzanow lies due south-west of Cracow. At the junction of Trzebinia on the direct line from Vienna they would be met by Bickmore in one or more of their three carriages and three pairs of horses, which Henry brought from England, and drive the three or four miles on to Chrzanow.

This was a typical Polish village, with a central market place from where the road led out to the Lowenfeld estate, and originally stopped at the main gates of the park. This abutted on the main road between Austria and Poland, and in due course Henry built a road out into the country beyond the village boundary, later to be known as the Heinrich Allee. Being Henry's creation, this was on the grand scale, with a double avenue of trees. Originally Rosa's stone house had been the only one in the enclosed park, but when the English family began to make their regular visits, Henry built the Gartenhaus for them, a one-storey dwelling leading on to the main drive. It had day and night nurseries, dining-room, morning and drawing-rooms, with bedroom and bath for the parents at one end. The nurseries looked on to a kitchen garden at the back, the first garden the girls had known. Beyond were the stables, and on a clear day they could see the Carpathians. Henry liked to play billiards, but Rosa had no table, so they made one on the estate and put it inside a specially designed building known as the 'Billiard House'.

All this was everything the children wanted, and the antithesis of everything they hated about London. All the cousins came in to the

Gartenhaus for the midday meal. At Chrzanow Nurse Minter's character underwent a sea change. She took charge of the foreign children with their uncouth—as she thought—ways, and took the family at face value in the Continental environment which she evidently enjoyed. Kasia, her predecessor at Lowndes Square who had originally come from Chrzanow, returned to Poland to become their cook. The children could run barefoot all over the estate, or they would drive in the mornings in a pony cart out into the forest, or to the lakes, by one of which the foresters had made a bathing place. If the family decided to picnic the head forester would make a large fire. Should their father be there at the time, the foresters would redouble their efforts for the master who had saved the estate, and would roast his favourite potatoes and anticipate his every wish.

Alice found life at Chrzanow boring compared with the social life in London, but she was interested in the local scene and helped the Jewish grocer enlarge and improve his stock. She relieved the monotony by importing house parties from England. Six bedrooms were added to the Gartenhaus, with a long veranda facing the main drive, and later other guest rooms for her friends. She and her guests could explore the tourist attraction of Zakopane in the mountains, a day-and-night trip on which Helena and Margaret did not accompany them, though they would go to Cracow and to the Castle Wawel where the Lowenfeld family silver could be admired in the museum. Helena remembered especially the salt mines of Wieliczka with their high roofs and stalactites and stalagmites which could be visited.

The peasants on the estate had a medieval relationship with the family. Helena was adopted by the villagers of Balin. It was her village, and though she later said she hated it, the women would kiss the hem of her skirt as she passed. She respected them, and all the people who worked on the estate, especially the 'garden girls' who tended the vegetables outside her nursery and the men who built the new road, infinitely preferring them to her mother's smart friends. Henry too was on good terms with his employees. When the railway was to be extended beyond Trzebinia he called the villagers to a gathering, at which he hoped to explain the mechanics of the steam locomotive which was to affect their lives. Helena remembered sitting beside him on the ground in front of the house with the men around him, as he drew the plan on the sandy soil. 'Thank you,' they said politely at the end of his talk. 'It was kind of you to explain it to us, but we feel sure there must be horses inside the engine.'

In Poland everything was as free as air and as natural. By contrast London was dull, solidly comfortable and life reasonably predictable. Alice had her social contacts, her musical afternoons, her seances and her dinner parties, none of which amused her children. They actively disliked some of her friends and hated being on show at her parties, where there was the ever-present risk of being kissed by strange women. On the other hand their father wanted them to see something of the outside world. Every 9 November he hired a window in Northumberland Avenue from where they could watch the Lord Mayor's procession. They saw Queen Victoria's Diamond Jubilee procession from a room overlooking the route, and in retrospect Helena remembered the Kaiser better than the Queen. Every Boxing Day Henry took his daughters to the pantomime at Drury Lane where they might see his great friend the comedian Dan Leno. Once the Apollo Theatre was in action a regular box was available for the family even if the performance was not always suitable.

Their father's friends were musicians, actors, writers and artists. Apart from Albeniz who came only to play the piano, the others came to Lowndes Square to talk. The girls were encouraged by their father to meet his friends and were prepared to listen happily to their conversation in any language. However, Henry failed to allow Helena to fulfil either of the two great ambitions of her childhood, to travel third class on a railway or to ride on the top of a horse bus. It was always the dreary, reserved first-class carriage by train, or their own horse-drawn carriages. In all other respects, though, Henry Lowenfeld was the father that every child would want, an amusing, lively, devoted extrovert.

However, Henry was at home less and less as time went on, and his marriage to Alice gradually deteriorated. The girls began to hear the word 'liaison' increasingly often muttered by their maternal aunts Edie and Flory, the latter an acidic spinster who was intensely loyal to Alice. Henry had evidently broken his word given to her at the time of their marriage that his mistresses would not impinge on the family life. The first reference to this appears in Margaret's diary in February 1898: 'Blowing up of trouble between M[other] and P[apa] re E D', an actress then playing at the Prince of Wales Theatre. She had heard her father say to her mother, 'If you don't like it, get out.'

On Helena the effect of the increasingly evident discord in the home may have been greater. She was later to write to her mother:

. . . Consider what a grotesque childhood we had; until I was 13, the word 'home' meant to me a place where my parents were incessantly fighting, the one swearing at the other, where nothing was secure, where we lived incessantly on the verge of a volcano.

HRW to AQ—Peking, 7.6.22

Early in 1898 a judicial separation was mooted; Alice's lawyers asked for a settlement of £1,500 a year for life, while Henry's lawyers proposed a figure of £500. In April the same year an entry in Margaret's diary reads: 'M and P reconciled,' but the reconciliation did not last. That year Rosa died, and Henry did not accompany his children on the regular summer holiday at Chrzanow. Instead the girls and their mother, taking 'Smuttles' with them, went to Poland via Rome, Hamburg and Berlin. They all, including Henry, spent the next Christmas in the new hotel he had bought and rebuilt in Sandown, and went back there the following summer. This time the girls, their mother and an assortment of her friends and relations stayed in Alice's villa, Bay View, while Henry stayed in the hotel. Significantly, so did his widowed Polish cousin, Frania Permutter. This pattern was repeated the following summer, but at Christmas Henry was at Lowndes Square for the family festivities. It was to be the last time.

The next year, having given Alice a diamond necklace for her birthday in July, Henry turned up in August at Chrzanow, where the family were staying. He brought with him Frania who remained for five days. Henry then drove her to the Russian border, came back, and asked Alice to divorce him so that he could marry Frania. Against Henry's wishes Alice went to Vienna, taking the girls with her for some reason, to discuss the Austrian divorce law with lawyers. She came back saying divorce would be a sin and she wanted Henry and herself to try once more to make the marriage work. Apparently Henry at first agreed, but then changed his mind. He had realised that a divorce would make him appear in the wrong so instead he started proceedings in Vienna to have the marriage annulled, declaring himself a Jew with Austrian nationality.

Meanwhile he suggested he should live with Frania at his hunting box at Aston Abbots, in England, and spend the holidays with Alice and his daughters. He even persuaded Alice to go to Warsaw to talk this extraordinary proposition over with Frania. Alice returned wounded and enraged from a fruitless mission, with the allegation that Frania was a 'wicked woman', and a gold-digger into the bargain. Frania was adamant that she intended to keep Henry to his promise to marry her. This is what he ultimately did, and in the end he treated Frania exactly as he had treated Alice by entering into a relationship with another woman. Although Helena for many years after the marriage refused to see Frania, she came eventually to realise that Frania really loved her father, and was far from being financially motivated. Helena described her changed views to her mother some twenty years later, after she had renewed their acquaintance-ship:

> You are wrong about Frania. I imagine that your estimate of her is now quite inaccurate. Life has punished her severely and she is a chastened person. Having started with your picture of her, I have gradually formed my own opinion, unbiased, and in many ways she has won my solid respect.
>
> HRW to AQ—Tsinan, 12.12.26

While the nullity proceedings were going through, Henry, accord-ing to Margaret, seems to have tried to explain things 'more or less' to his children, but without much success. On 30 October 1901, she noted in her diary, 'I write my mind to P'. It was the mind of a miser-able eleven-year-old. In the same month Henry told Alice he would be bringing Frania to Lowndes Square for Christmas and Alice was to move out of the house. Accordingly she and the girls went to relations for Christmas, and when they returned to Lowndes Square Henry had left for the last time.

That winter Alice's health was in worse shape than usual, and in February she was operated on, as was the custom of the day, in her own home at Lowndes Square, by the distinguished surgeon at the Middlesex Hospital, Sir John Bland-Sutton, then at the peak of his career. Alice's previous ill health and the prospect of her operation caused Helena much anxiety which she expressed in a letter from school. It contains incidentally the first reference to her belief in an afterlife, this at the age of thirteen.

> Does Papa know he won't have us? Are we proper wards of Chancery now? And will we live with Auntie Bea [her mother's sister]? . . . Now Goodbye my darling Mother. This may be the last letter I shall write to you and I may never see you again in

this world, but I hope and pray that I may . . . If possible come back and tell me what the next world is like.
From you ever-loving
Ellie

HRW to AL—9.2.02

And then on 12 February:

Just heard the operation is over. I am *so* pleased. I *told* you so. I *knew* you wouldn't die. O my duck I feel so happy . . . this is a sign that all this trouble will end happily or else you wouldn't be allowed to live.
Goodbye darling from your own loving joyful
Ellie

HRW to AL—12.2.02

Helena had had permission, previously withheld by Alice, to write to her father about her mother's operation and thought it did some good; 'If kindness won't do for the man he must have plain speaking, and goodness knows I gave him little enough of it.' She thought her letter had been useful as Henry had stayed at his country house all the morning in order to be telegraphed 'the minute the operation was over'. 'Now if I hadn't he would not perhaps have known of it.'

Four weeks later Margaret's diary of 13 March 1902 tells us, 'M downstairs. Vienna suit heard.' Alice had contested the latter on the plea that Henry, far from being an Austrian Jew, had been baptised in the Roman Catholic faith of his mother and was domiciled in England. She even toyed with the idea of becoming a Catholic herself. Her lawyers were unsuccessful, however, and the marriage was dissolved by the proper court in Vienna which accepted that the husband had Austrian domicile—he had in fact been back to Austria every year since he left in order to maintain these rights.

After the Vienna verdict without further warning Henry and Frania were married the following month at a registry office in London on 18 April 1902. The first Helena and Margaret knew of this event was from their aunts, who had read the announcement in the papers. The furore this created in London can be imagined. Henry had committed bigamy, no less, in the eyes of Alice and her family, and Alice immediately instigated proceedings for divorce in London in order to establish her daughters' legitimacy and protect her own position.

The hearing, in July 1902, lasted six days. Alice had applied for the case to be tried by a special jury and not in open court. The Registrar refused the application, but Alice successfully appealed against this. Henry then appealed against the decision of the Court of Appeal for the hearing to be re-argued in open court but this was dismissed without a judgement. Alice having established the validity of her English marriage, the divorce finally went through that autumn. Alice was left with a large settlement, a capital sum to bring her in £200 a month, the house and custody of the two girls.

The consequences were, of course, far reaching. Apart from the immediate effect of the family break-up on the girls, Helena has said that her father's treatment of her mother was the driving incentive which led her later to devote her professional life to the interests of women. It was a painful evolution, because as her letters showed, she also became intensely critical of her mother. Aided and abetted by her own family Alice taught her daughters to despise their father, as evidenced by this letter from Helena to her mother:

> . . . I was allowed to think of my father as a person impossible to respect, a person guilty of nearly every possible beastliness. Just think for a minute what a profound violation of the simplest rights of childhood that means, and what a bad effect a life like that, lasting 14 years, must have had on both our minds.
>
> HRW to AQ—Peking, 12.12.22

Helena's dislike for her father was so fostered that once, before the divorce, when riding in the Park, she met her father driving in his phaeton with Frania and tried to hit him with her whip. He then threatened to take Helena out of Alice's charge. Alice went hotfoot to the Public Prosecutor but was powerless in view of the Vienna verdict. Helena, however, remained with her mother and on increasingly bad terms with her father. After one meeting when she went specially to see him in Bath, accompanied by 'Smuttles', she returned saying she had finished with him for good. A letter to 'My darling Mama' illustrates the young Helena's implacable resentment:

> If Papa is going to propose that we should live with him just say he can save himself the trouble in my case, as it will be quite as much as I can manage to even treat him as a human being and not like the *Devil* he is. Auntie Bea wrote saying he threatened to prove us illegitimate, *nice* sort of thing to do to your children . . .

Now Goodnight my poor wee darling. Wait just a week and I'll be at home to cheer you up. It's a pity you can't marry me and *roast* that *Devil*.

HRW to AL—25.3.02

That Christmas Henry sent Margaret presents, including a bay hunter by the name of Robin—Margaret enjoyed hunting, unlike Helena —but gave Helena nothing.

Relations between Henry and Alice became so petty that shortly after the divorce his lawyers wrote to say that Mr Lowenfeld wanted to know if his former wife wished him to raise his hat to her should they meet in the street. He would have done better if he could have come to some agreement with Alice whereby he could remain on good terms at least with his daughters, but the concept was never presented to the girls that the affairs of husband and wife are their own business and nothing to do with the children, whose duty is to remain friendly to both. After the divorce the girls were forbidden—though they asked to do so many times—even to write to their father, let alone see him, which Helena later believed did great harm to two sensitive children. There is no doubt that this contributed to Helena's great initial prejudice against her father. Confronted with her mother's vocal and reiterated complaints, 'My own little darling', she wrote to her from school:

> *When* are you going to learn sense? You ought to jump for joy at getting Papa out of the house. You can't possibly miss him, that's all rot. You are really relieved, my beauty. Anyway I am much nicer than he so you won't miss him when I am at home.
>
> HRW to AL—6.11.01

Her attempts at comforting her mother had not been particularly successful when she urged her 'own little darling' to 'cheer up' with these crumbs:

> There is one comfort. You are having such a bad time in this world you will have a heavenly time in the next when we poor creatures are languishing in our little mists. Think what an amount of punishment Papa will get. I *am* sorry for him, poor man.
>
> HRW to AL—3.11.01

[4]

Life Without Father

'It is awfully good of you to let me have another chance,' wrote Helena to her mother, when she was finally allowed to leave Miss Glatz's school and go to Cheltenham Ladies' College. 'I am really grateful and will try to get on there. I hope I shan't make a mess of that school.' Margaret remained with Alice for another year in Lowndes Square after Henry's departure, and then joined Helena at Cheltenham in the same boarding-house, Bunwell.

Cheltenham transformed Helena's life. She had a room of her own, the food was good, and there were few rules. For the first time in her life she enjoyed lessons. Twenty years later she wrote to her mother:

> I shall always be endlessly grateful to you for sending me to Cheltenham where my mind was stimulated, tastes opened out, and where my splendid friends, especially the elder ones, took infinite trouble to give me just the training that my home had been unable to do . . . When I went to the College . . . for the first time I felt my power, and really enjoyed myself. It was a glorious discovery to find that I was stronger than most people there and could make the other girls do as I liked. Of course my undisciplined erratic childhood bore fruit, and I was absolutely unruly—but that was nothing, a natural reaction after years of most unnatural environment.
>
> HRW to AQ—Peking, 7.6.22

Helena was at Cheltenham at the same time as Lucy Wills, destined too to be distinguished in the field of medicine—as a haematologist and nutritionist who gave her name to an essential food factor and to a disease. Helena was later to meet her again as a young student at the Royal Free Hospital. Both came under the influence at Cheltenham of one of the great pioneers of women's education, Dorothea Beale. In the middle of the nineteenth century Dorothea Beale, with Frances Mary Buss, who had been her schoolmate and was later headmistress

43

of the North London Collegiate School, laid bare the shortcomings of women's education. Miss Buss will be remembered for her immortal remark: 'Now what I say is: Why did the Lord create Huntley and Palmer to make cakes [sic] for us if not to give our clever girls a chance to do something better?'

By the time Helena arrived at the College Miss Beale had been its Principal for over forty years. She had been chosen from fifty candidates in 1857 when there were only sixty-nine pupils. She raised Cheltenham to the forefront of English girls' schools; it had ten boarding-houses and, at the time of her death in 1906, nearly a thousand girls, Helena among them, went by train to her funeral in Gloucester Cathedral.

Oliver (Tom) Hill was still the only boy of Helena's own age in her circle, and her father the only man. At Ealing her friends, including Ina the head girl, were older than herself. She followed the same pattern at Cheltenham. She was attracted by a young assistant house mistress—'the first adult to excite my admiration'—and she cultivated an intellectual relationship with Miss Margery Reid, a teacher who was in charge of the College museum and whose father had been a contemporary of both Darwin and Wallace. She had been brought up on their arguments about the nature of evolution, which had set her mind on scientific lines, and she was interested in butterflies, minerals and flowers. Helena described her later as a female Dan Leno, a short woman with a humorous face. Helena helped her in the museum with the catalogue which she was reorganising, and on Saturdays she would help Margery Reid in her own garden. Gardening, to which she was thus introduced for the first time, was to remain a major interest throughout her life.

Meanwhile in Lowndes Square Alice was on the downward slope from unlimited to limited riches, and decided to move the one-parent family to Cheltenham so that the girls could live at home instead of boarding at Bunwell House. She bought Oakfield House to which she moved shortly after Henry and Frania's marriage. It had a large garden, three vineries, a peach house and tennis court. Alice took with her to Cheltenham everything from Lowndes Square, all the dining-room, morning room, drawing-room and study furniture, including the billiard table. She then devoted herself to establishing the same sort of social round she had enjoyed in London. The move did not please Helena, who had not been consulted and resented it. She had no interest in the Primrose League, and would not even help her mother when the latter took to growing mushrooms in the cellar and keeping bees in the garden in the new house.

'Smuttles' came with them to Oakfield, adding a sense of continuity and security. There were no lessons in the afternoon in Miss Beale's day, and the girls came home at midday, and only went back to the College in the afternoon for games, or extras, which in Helena's case were music lessons and some drawing classes. She never liked living in Cheltenham, much preferring London, and told her mother so in the flood of letters she later wrote home from China. It says much for Alice that she kept all her daughters' letters, however critical, for posterity.

Darling Mother,
. . . For my part, I hated going away [from London], I knew I should never belong to Cheltenham, and always intended to get back to London as soon as possible, the place had no interest for me whatever, except College and my College friends . . . Of course I loved the house and garden, but never looked on it as a permanency, because I knew I could never feel at home in a little gossipy country town. That our home life there failed was, I think, due to two main reasons, one that you do not understand young people, their inevitable egotism, their independent development, and their varying needs, and so we were continually puzzling you and annoying you; second that the emphasis in your own mind about the important things in the home was wrong.

You expected *us* to make up to *you* for *your* marriage troubles, and you thought we ought to be interested in making the home bright and so on, for you. Now, in the name of impersonal common sense, why on earth should the children make up to the mother for a mistake in marriage made before they were born? Rather the other way round—your troubles were in no sense our fault. They were grievous, but they were your own affair.

It was literally *impossible* for me to be interested in the Primrose League, or your social struggles. It wasn't in me. You made a fatal mistake when I began to find my own friends. You disliked them and showed plainly that you were jealous of them. I got so used to your being always hurt or annoyed about something that it became the normal atmosphere between us. Of course circumstances were against us. By the time I was 15 or 16, it was evident that my character was stronger than yours, that was neither of our faults, but it made it very difficult for both of us.

HRW to AQ—Peking, 17.6.22

But poor Alice had one redeeming feature which Helena recognised and for which she was ever grateful—Alice was an inveterate traveller. She provided for her children holidays in Europe and America, to places which most tourists hardly ever visited at that time. When Helena was sixteen Alice asked her if she would like to go on a Hellenic cruise to Greece, Egypt, Italy and Palestine, the latter then still under Ottoman rule. In the spring of 1904 the two of them sailed on the ss *Argonaut* from the London docks, first stop Jaffa, now part of Tel Aviv. The sea was rough and they were rowed ashore to find huge baskets of Jaffa oranges, which Helena had never before tasted, at the equivalent of 6d a basket. On by train to Jerusalem, over a plain covered with small red anemones, the Rose of Sharon. The train travelled so slowly that the thirty-five-mile journey took three hours, and Helena, who jumped off to gather anemones, caught it up on foot.

In Jerusalem she shared a bedroom with her mother in a primitive hotel outside the Damascus Gate. It had no bathroom but one tap and a basin in a cupboard in the passage. She recalled that in this hotel she ate an omelette made from an ostrich egg, and that it was very good. Other memories were of the Via Dolorosa to the Church of the Holy Sepulchre.

It was the year in which Helena was confirmed: 'I was more or less a Christian by then, but I never believed for a moment that Calvary could have been where the Church stands.' General Charles Gordon, visiting Jerusalem in 1883, became convinced that the true burial place of Jesus was in the cave known as Gordon's Calvary in the Garden of Joseph of Arimathea, and Helena concurred.

She had a psychic impression of tragedy in the Garden of Gethsemane and the Mount of Olives. Thence to Jericho, where the travel organisers had bribed the strongest bandits to guard their horse carriages from lesser bandits. From the hills above she saw the Dead Sea, looking blue and beautiful like any other sea, but found it no fun and even dangerous to swim in the salt water.

In Egypt she climbed a pyramid and reached the top ahead of the others, from where she could see the green strip of the Nile in miles and miles of desert. Each step of the pyramid was a cubic yard and each tourist had two Arab guides. 'Missie, you climb like a wild gazelle,' her guardians told her. Thence by camel to the Sphinx, without her mother, but with the two Arabs. 'Please come home with me and be my wife,' said one. It was the sixteen-year-old girl's first proposition.

Even before the end of the next school term Alice was off again, this time with both girls, and Miss Beale's permission, for three months. They were sitting at breakfast one morning reading the papers when Alice raised her head and said, 'Girls, I see there is to be a World Exhibition in St Louis this summer. You'd like to see America, wouldn't you?' They would and they did. Alice fixed up a tour with Thomas Cook in which they would concentrate on the natural phenomena of America rather than its cities. Accordingly they left Liverpool on 2 July 1904 on the Cunarder s s *Devonia* for Boston. The fare for each passenger travelling first class was £13; the journey took nine days.

From Boston they went by train to New York where in the Broadway Hotel they were surprised to learn from the bellboy that their shoes would be stolen if they left them outside their bedroom doors to be cleaned. More surprisingly the same bellboy brought a message from another guest in the hotel that he would like to buy their hats. When the offer was refused, he raised his price, but without any luck. Of St Louis, the object ostensibly of the expedition, Helena remembered little, except that the temporary exhibition buildings, when they arrived there on 16 July, seemed excessively hot. In Salt Lake City Helena found the lake as disagreeable to swim in as the Dead Sea. Being Helena she soon entered into an altercation with the Mormons. They were distinctly less complimentary than her Arab contacts. One told her that were she the last woman in the world he would not marry her.

Alice proved an intrepid traveller. She hired three mules on which they descended along the narrow zig-zag trail eighteen inches wide in places, seven miles down from the rim of the Grand Canyon to the base of the gorge, going back a million years in time for every twenty feet in height. The varying orange to mauve colours of shales, sandstone and limestone exposed in layers over 500 million years entranced Helena. The heat reflected off the sloping sides was intense, and they were glad of the hats which had attracted so much attention in New York. Alice began to show signs of sunstroke and Helena dipped her handkerchief in the Colorado River to cool her mother's forehead, but it dried in four seconds.

A five-day journey by stage coach to the Yellowstone Park followed. There, brown bears were indigenous, and there they watched while the fish caught in the lake were cooked in the boiling water of a raised geyser. Thence by train up the west coast through Pasadena, Los Angeles, Santa Barbara and San Francisco to the Yosemite Valley. After exploring by coach the natural wonders, the lake and the falls, they retraced their way home over the Rockies on the Canadian Pacific Railway, through Banff and past the Great Lakes. In the observation coach Helena encountered a geographer who was engaged in finding appropriate names for as yet unidentified peaks. He asked Helena if she had any suitable ideas—he had been through the Old Testament and kings of England, but had no more suggestions. For once Helena was flummoxed, but not for long. She came out with 'Kipling'. Rudyard Kipling (1865–1936) was then one of her heroes. The *Jungle* books (1894 and 1895) had been among her childhood favourites and *Kim* (1901) and *Just So Stories* (1902) were recent additions to her reading. After his years in India Kipling had married the sister of an American friend and they lived for a while in Vermont. History does not relate if it is anything to do with Helena, but today there happens to be a town by the name of Kipling in Saskatchewan, fifteen miles south of the CPR line.

Only one train on this historic Lowenfeld journey arrived on time, and at Lake Louise they waited twenty-four hours for a 'lost' train. Another caught fire. A cloudburst in Arizona was so violent that the tracks were buried in sand. After what seemed an interminable delay, Helena went to investigate. She offered to clear the track if the driver would lend her a spade, which he did. The idea had not occurred to the other travellers, who then came forward to help and together they got the train going again. In spite of these set-backs they finally arrived, via Calgary, Niagara, Toronto, and Quebec, in Liverpool on 28 September 1903, only two weeks late for the autumn term at Cheltenham. It had been a journey from which the young Helena retained vivid memories of the natural beauties of America.

A courier at Thomas Cook's had made out the North American itinerary. Every year thereafter this enterprising man organised unusual holidays off the beaten track for Alice and her family. Once it was Portugal—in the last year of the monarchy—then Denmark, Corsica, Norway, including an island in the Christiana (now Oslo) Fjord, Italy, France, and Sweden, where Helena saw, and enjoyed, organised segregated nude bathing for the first time.

Alice, who was a chronic invalid, even perhaps a hypochondriac, in England was indomitable abroad. Margaret Lowenfeld's notes, compiled from her diary, contain many references to her mother's ill health, although this did not significantly affect the programme as described:

August 1905. Up the Swedish coast by train, boat and driving to Stockholm. Mother ill—recovered. I chased in street. To Straalsund Rugen. Mother ill. Great difficulty feeding her.

1 January 1907. Berlin to Cracow. Heavy snow, arrived 11 p.m. instead of 8 p.m. Two sleighs to Hotel Dresden.

2 January 1907. M not well and stayed in bed. Lunch Hotel Saxe. M ill and back to hotel.

4 January 1907. To Chrzanow to take wreath to family grave. 3.15 Trzebinia to Vienna. Arrived 11 p.m.

8 January 1907. Back to Berlin.

10 January 1907. To Flushing and Queensborough by night.

11 January 1907. Up 5 a.m. Arrived Victoria 8 a.m. To Paddington and Cheltenham. Mother and Helena to Hunt Ball that night. Back 3 a.m.

The divorce had not affected the holidays in Poland, and the contacts with the Lowenfeld cousins were uninterrupted. Helena and Margaret continued to visit their uncle Willi, the judge in Berlin. For Helena this meant that for one mark she could sit nightly on the floor with other students and enjoy the Berlin Philharmonic concerts. These cosmopolitan and educational pleasures which Alice instigated were duly acknowledged by Helena, but it is questionable if they compensated for her mother's alleged personality defects, which strained relations between mother and daughter. If Alice disliked Helena's school friends, as her daughter contended, and did not invite them to Oakfield, both girls loathed their mother's men friends. They particularly resented two men, Frank Quicke, whom Alice later married, and Billy Taylor, who had both been on the scene before the divorce. Helena described them as 'intolerable and repulsive puss cats who sit around in women's drawing-rooms'. Her antipathy is expressed in extracts from a letter she wrote to her mother many years later:

Darling Mother

. . . I have for some time thought it might help you to understand me and our relationship if I took the trouble to tell you the story of our life together . . . from my point of view, which I don't think you have ever contemplated. I must begin by saying two things, one that I fully and freely agree with you that I am a rotten daughter, that, in fact, I understand very little about being a daughter, and second that this recital is in no sense a grievance, nor a complaint against anyone, it is simply an account of the facts as they appear to me . . .

The time of the divorce was an epoch . . . By that time there was one thing about you which worried me considerably, and that was your men friends. Your taste very early seemed to me, to put it politely, peculiar. Either you did not know a bounder when you saw one, or you enjoyed their society. I never decided which. Your friends who were constantly at Lowndes Square, Frank and Mr Taylor both . . . made me feel sick. I could not, and cannot, imagine how you can endure either of them for an hour. Then there was Maddick, ugh—he hung around endlessly, to everyone's disgust but yours. The worst of all was that creature Cordell in Hamburg—do you know that the way you behaved with him made me so ashamed that I used to wonder if I ought to write and tell my father—I was a very observant child and there was nothing I didn't notice. Even when I boiled over and hit the man in public you didn't realise what a severe blow you were dealing to my respect for you—you put it off by saying that I was jealous; so I was, of your good name, not in the way you thought. I tell you this now, because that train of thought had a strong influence in my relationship to you, which I don't think you realised at all. The man disappeared when we left the place, as his kind do, and you thought that was all . . .

HRW to AQ—Peking, 7.6.22

Frank Quicke's presence at Oakfield continually irked both Margaret and Helena who believed him to be a gold-digger. He stayed at Cheltenham on and off as soon as Alice moved there, and there are numerous references to him in Margaret's diary. About one of her mother's parties she wrote:

24 May 1906. Mother's Reception. Frank came . . . and won a prize. His friend told him 'the woman is evidently in love with you', but advised the time was not ripe for an offer.

The following year, shortly after their return from a Polish holiday, Frank evidently decided the time *was* ripe:

15–19 January 1907. Frank staying. He talked to Helena *re* marrying Mother. She to me. Both felt that if they wanted it we had no right to interfere. Frank back to London.

30 January 1907. Mother to town. He proposed to her. She refused.

31 January 1907. Tom [Hill] said Frank would insist on marrying her. Sad letter from Frank. This made her write and wire repeatedly asking him to come and stay in Cheltenham. [He was in a bad way financially, just recovered from a long illness and was homeless.]

2 February 1907. Frank arrived 9.30.

3 February 1907. Kept my birthday [actual birthday 2 February]. Frank kissed M and announced their engagement. Later asked M to marry him at once and she refused. He rushed out of the house without hat or coat. M in fearful state of nerves. Later Frank back and Helena pacified him. That night Mother very unhappy. Came to my room and took me in to sleep with her and said she did not want to marry Frank. I too tired to take much in. Very confused.

The upshot was that Alice and Frank were married in London ten weeks later. Maddened as she was by Frank Quicke, Helena admitted that he had the ability to make her mother feel wanted after all her years of loneliness before and after the divorce. He was gentle, solicitous and kind to her. At last she had become the centre of someone's attention. After their marriage they went to India for two months and their return from this protracted honeymoon was the beginning of an unhappy period for Helena, and for Margaret. In her later letters from China Helena made it clear that she was increasingly out of sympathy with her mother during this era:

The divorce . . . stimulated my loyalty to you a great deal. I think it was during the years in Cheltenham that we drifted furthest apart, and I think I understand now, more or less why it was. If you have patience I will try to explain.

You had a theory that you went there entirely for our sakes and that we therefore ought to be very grateful to you, and that you entered on your social battles there for our sakes. Your social battles made me smile even then. Why couldn't you realise that you were doing it for yourself to re-establish your own feeling of a place in the community? A social position anywhere means nothing to me, and never did. I'm like my father in that . . .

HRW to AQ—Peking, 7.6.22

There is less documentary evidence about the relationship between Alice and her younger daughter at this time. We do know that when Margaret was approaching sixteen, the age when she could legally choose between her divorced parents, she refused her father's invitation to go and live with him. However, she had her troubles at Cheltenham and recorded bleakly in her diary:

9 October 1905. I break down. To Dr Cargill. She says one month without school work.
20 October 1905. P sends £100 for a journey for me.
23 October 1905. P sends me £23. I write to him.
26 October 1905. I alone to see Dr Cargill. *My first move of revolt.*

Travel was Alice's panacea, and a few days later she and Margaret were off on RMS *Trent* for a tour of the West Indies, bound for Barbados, Trinidad, Puerto Columbia, Panama and Jamaica. They were back in time for Christmas. Perhaps the journey was therapeutic, but trouble was to recur.

After Alice's marriage to Frank Quicke the unpleasantness began in earnest at Oakfield. There were constant arguments with Frank, with Alice in tears much of the time. The rows seem to have been mainly between Margaret and Frank Quicke as Margaret recorded:

2 January 1908. Long discussion with M. She said I rude. Frank furious.
16 January 1908. Row between Frank and I. He exceedingly rude. General upset. M ill. I apologised in the end for peace. M crying most of the time.

And so it went on. Margaret had increasing nightmares. Meanwhile at the end of term examinations Helena found she could understand nothing in the arithmetic paper on her desk. She could make no sense of the figures which danced around the page. She was sent home, and was indeed on the verge of a mental breakdown. She consulted at her own insistence a woman doctor, Frances Stoney, who tried to get over to Alice that in her view the girls should live away from home. It was useless. Alice would not accept this and constantly accused her daughters of wanting to leave her. Frank did not help matters by telling her she must choose between him and them. Taylor was their intermediary but he achieved nothing constructive in the melodrama, only further aggravation.

The news reached Henry Lowenfeld, who came to the rescue. After much argument with Alice he arranged six months' respite. He rented 'Sultanpore' for his daughters, a house with a small garden at Little Brickhill. It was on the main road, on the Woburn estate, and close to the woods where there were wild lilies of the valley and where the current Duchess of Bedford, an ex-Cheltenham girl popularly known as the 'Flying Duchess', let them roam at will. It was the perfect temporary solution to their problems. By now Helena had gradually begun to review her opinion of her father as an entirely despicable individual. But owing to what she later described as 'adolescent narrow mindedness' she could not yet bring herself to meet Frania, whom she still blamed for the divorce.

Henry was living with Frania in another large London house in Hyde Park Square, but neither Margaret nor Helena would go there, 'which in his broadmindedness Papa accepted'. If they wished to see their father the girls went to his office, though such visits were infrequent and contrary to Alice's wishes. Cheltenham remained 'home' in spite of Frank's presence.

From Helena's and Margaret's point of view their father's idea of a temporary release for them was little short of a miracle. His proposition was unbelievably successful. At Little Brickhill Smuttles and the two girls lived happily on their own, cared for by village servants in great comfort miles from anywhere, with a horse, Giant, a pony carriage, Papa's cash and one of Papa's motors to use as they wished. They asked whoever they wished to stay, including Cheltenham friends; they went up to London, or back to Cheltenham as the mood took them. Two or three times a week their father came over from his house at Aston Abbots. Helena's heart was filled and comforted by the peace and beauty around. As she wrote to Alice:

Never again can you say that I'm only happy in a life of excitement. Absolutely nothing happens here, and I'm as happy as a Greek. There is never enough time for all the things I want to get done. I *love*, *adore* and *revel* in the pine woods.

HRW to AQ—Sultanpore, 3.2.08

The habit of letter writing was deeply ingrained and mother and daughter wrote to each other several times a week when separated. Alice's letters at this stage were apt to consist of a string of complaints. She had become soured and unforgiving and Helena had not yet developed an immunity to her mother's recriminations. Her letters to Alice were invariably affectionate.

'Darling Mother,' she wrote once during the Little Brickhill interlude, 'You can't think how happy it made me to get a *happy* letter from you.' Happy letters from Alice were rare occurrences. She had taken badly to the whole Little Brickhill relief operation, and expressed her dissatisfaction in a string of complaints. Helena had shown no remorse on leaving home. She had sent her mother a wire for her wedding anniversary when flowers would have been in order. She had given Frank the impression of being conscious of her own superiority, and so on.

Alice's resentment against Henry for bringing the nullity suit had grown with the years, but contact with her father and the passage of time had induced in Helena another view of the past, and now she replied to Alice's continued reference to the suit:

My darling Mother

How can you bring up that nullity suit again? Where is your Christian forgiveness? If it had come off the injury to us would have been much more cruel than to you, because you could have married again, but the stain would have been upon us all our lives. We have fully forgiven Papa long ago (never mind whether it was difficult or not). Now that does not mean in any degree that we condone the idea or loathe it less, but simply that I have tried to act on what we understand of God's forgiveness to us. Apart from that I think there's a good deal of misconception about that part of the case, but that doesn't affect my forgiveness. So Mother can't you forgive too?

HRW to AQ—Sultanpore, 13.2.08

This led only to further argument as to the rights and wrongs committed several years earlier. As for her father's authority, Helena assured her mother that Henry would not spare his daughters when he saw their faults. He had already drawn Helena's attention to her innate lack of tact. Alice remained unconvinced but some sort of agreement was reached and eventually both girls and Smuttles returned to Cheltenham refreshed in spirit.

It was their last year at Cheltenham. Helena was due to go to medical school that autumn. She had enjoyed life at the College and earned Miss Beale's approval as to her general conduct although occasionally, as her reports indicate, 'more quiet application' was to be desired. Her house mistress also found her conduct 'very good' and considered Helena an 'intelligent and responsive pupil'. Again, 'more gentleness and quietness of manner' was evidently desirable. She left with many friends among the staff. She had remained good at Euclid, but her scholastic record had not been distinguished. She had failed to matriculate at the first attempt in 1906, but passed the second time. The qualities which made her such a good doctor—her independent outlook and her many outside interests—did not make a good candidate for examinations. '*Don't* make up the answers this time, Ellie,' her form mistress had instructed her as she personally escorted her to the door of the examination room when she re-sat her Latin paper.

She could have gone to medical school earlier, but she had stayed on at Cheltenham Ladies' College until she was twenty in order to take the first medical examination at school. Helena was the only student who was taking the Preliminary Science course in Physics and Chemistry, and she enjoyed the undivided attention of a teacher, Miss Agatha Leonard, whom she greatly admired. Miss Leonard's testimonial appears on Helena Rosa Lowenfeld's application for admittance to the London (Royal Free Hospital) School of Medicine for Women, dated 11 June 1908. Miss Leonard stated that she had known the applicant for four years. This document remains in the Royal Free Hospital archives. With Pre-Sci behind her Helena could go straight into the second year of the medical course at the School of Medicine, which she entered in October 1908, to be followed two years later by Margaret.

After Helena left the College, Alice sold Oakfield and bought a house at Hounslow, which was to be their next home. Until the move was completed Helena lived temporarily with Alice's sister in Sloane Street in order to begin her medical studies in London. Her aunt was

married to a surgeon at St George's Hospital with whom Frank
Quicke managed to have arguments—as well as with his stepdaugh-
ters. Margaret remained with her mother and her misery continued:

> *1 October 1908.* Dr Stoney tries to negotiate with M that H and I
> should live alone. Useless. M weeps. Endless discussions with
> M about our going to P's office. Dr S tells M I must get away
> from my family. I continue to have nightmares.

Predictably, Alice decided to follow her usual procedure and took
her daughter Margaret abroad. They went to Berlin three weeks later
where, after a few days, Alice left Margaret in order to return to
Frank. From England she proceeded to write and wire about future
plans. Henry Lowenfeld wanted Margaret to stay in Berlin and
eventually Alice grudgingly agreed, at least until after Christmas. In
order to smooth things over, Clara, Willi Lowenfeld's wife, invited
Frank and Alice for Christmas, but Alice said she was not well enough
to go, and only Helena went briefly to Berlin. In the New Year Alice
arrived to fetch Margaret home and the Berlin Lowenfelds tried to
persuade her to let the girls live alone, but to no effect. Margaret
returned with her mother to London, Alice having extracted from her
a promise that she would stay with her for at least a year, and not see
her father during this period. Alice was unable, and did not even try,
to prevent her elder daughter from seeing her father during this year,
but she asked both girls for 'a little sacrifice' in a letter addressed to
'The Misses Lowenfeld'. Alice begged that:

> She [Helena] will not publicly identify herself in any way with
> her father by going to his office or any public entertainment with
> him. After the year she can do exactly as she wishes . . . Had
> your father behaved in a gentlemanly manner and was willing to
> do so in the future I would not have asked such a promise. At the
> end of the year Madge also to be released of all duty to me and
> decide for herself what she wishes to do. During this year I beg
> both my children not to allow their father to speak or write
> disrespectfully of me or my family.
> Your loving Mother
> A Q to H R W and M L—Oakfield, 29.6.08

Helena came of age on 17 September that year. She spent her
twenty-first birthday with her father, who took a suite at Claridge's.
They had meals in their private sitting-room, in deference perhaps to

Alice's wishes. Henry filled it with flowers and inundated Helena with gifts, a fox fur, jewellery and a tortoiseshell dressing-table set. The gift Helena cherished most was a pearl bracelet which had belonged to her grandmother. The identical bracelet had been discovered at Rosa's death to consist of artificial pearls. It transpired that when the Chrzanow estate fell on hard times Rosa had sold her bracelet to a Paris jeweller who made a copy using the original rose-diamond and pearl clasp. After her death when the secret was discovered Henry collected carefully matched genuine pearls to replace the artificial ones, so that Helena might have her grandmother's reconstructed bracelet for her twenty-first birthday. He extracted from her a promise that she would never sell or give it away. The original had been a double strand and Margaret had a similar bracelet when she came of age.

After Alice's move to London, while Helena and Margaret were living with her at Hounslow, both girls fell out regularly with Frank Quicke, who was often drunk, although Alice appeared indifferent to or oblivious of his excessive drinking. The saga is continued by Margaret who noticed that the strain was beginning to tell on Helena, while she herself was now prone to attacks of vomiting:

> *12 March 1909.* Row between F and H. F departs to Taylor's flat and writes to M he won't come back. She goes and fetches him back.
> *14 March 1909.* Scene evening between F and M about us. Taylor to negotiate.
> *15 March 1909.* F capitulates.
> *29 October 1909.* I seem to have spent a good deal of this time being ill and in bed.
> *4 December 1909.* I fainted in the skating rink.

Helena had her own troubles. She found the journey to the medical school long and tedious. Later she admitted to a nagging fear, even a phobia, that she would fall on the line at Hounslow West whence she travelled daily to Russell Square. She had a compulsive urge to hold on to the wall at the back of the platform, before boarding the train. It was against this unhappy background that Helena embarked on her medical career.

[5]

Embryo Doctor

Helena entered the London School of Medicine for Women on the threshold of a career which she had decided to follow when she was six years old. It was an intention from which she had never deviated. No clear reason emerges as to why the little girl announced her decision at her mother's luncheon table in the presence of a visitor. She had no medical relatives, and at the time no personal experience of doctors other than those who attended her little sister for a series of minor ailments. 'Baby' seemed always to be ill, but this was more a source of irritation than of serious anxiety in the Lowenfeld household. Helena always maintained that her profession was written in her stars.

Alice had presented her elder daughter at Court when Helena was eighteen, an experience which intrigued Helena, who fell in with her mother's arrangements, and donned the statutory feathers and train, which took some manipulating, to curtsy before Edward VII and Queen Alexandra, the memory of whose porcelain face remained vividly imprinted. She was impressed with the organisation by which all the girls in trains and feathers were given an excellent supper at the Palace after their presentation. The whole performance threw an interesting light, she thought, on the lives of royalty. She remained sceptical, however, of the merits of her mother's reasoning that henceforth she would be accepted at any court in Europe.

Whatever social expectations Alice may have had for her daughters, she had provided for them a first-class education, and made no objection to Helena's choice of career. Her father had smiled indulgently on the idea and it was only later that Helena learnt that Henry Lowenfeld had considerable difficulty in adjusting to the idea that he had two modern daughters bent on following a profession. He had hoped they would marry into the world of banking, and he was not familiar with career women, let alone women doctors, although he had heard that Dr Cargill had been involved with Margaret's health and knew that Helena had expressly asked for a woman doctor during her mental breakdown. It was not a common profession for women at the beginning of the century and there were still obstacles to be overcome in their training.

Until 1886 when the Edinburgh school opened its doors, the medical school to which Helena now went daily was the only one in the United Kingdom which would accept women students. As a 'fresher' in 1908 Helena would have seen the plaque in the Common Room which reads, 'The London School of Medicine for Women was established in August 1874 through the efforts of Miss Sophia Jex-Blake, MD'. Sophia Jex-Blake's struggle for women's medical education had been an uphill one. Under the Medical Act of 1511 both men and women could practise medicine unrestrictedly in London or within seven miles of its walls, provided they were licensed after examination by the Bishop of London and the Dean of St Paul's with the aid of competent doctors of physic as assessors. Anyone could get on the Register formed by the 1858 Medical Registration Act if holding a diploma, or degree granted by a recognised examining body, but all the nineteen examining bodies in the United Kingdom refused to examine women candidates. Elizabeth Garrett managed to qualify in 1865 by taking the examination of the Society of Apothecaries (LSA), the only body from which women were then not totally barred. Four years later the Apothecaries closed this loophole by altering their charter, and in 1865 women were specifically excluded by statute from the Medical Register unless they were already graduates of a recognised foreign university. Dr Elizabeth Blackwell held the distinction of being the first woman to gain admittance to the British Register. She had emigrated to America, then much more liberal than Britain towards medical women, had qualified in medicine and returned to England. Until 1869 she and Elizabeth Garrett were the only two registered women doctors practising in the United Kingdom.

Unable to gain admittance to any other school Sophia Jex-Blake successfully applied in 1869 to the University of Edinburgh, and with six other women matriculated in the Faculty of Medicine, only to be thwarted by the board of the Infirmary, which obstinately refused to let them on the wards. The indomitable Sophia decided to form her own medical school, and was determined to persuade a hospital to give her students the necessary clinical training.

She set up the London School of Medicine for Women in a small two-storeyed Georgian house in Bloomsbury, 30 Henrietta Street, renamed Handel Street in 1888 by the Metropolitan Board of Works. The house had at one time been occupied by Mrs Fitzherbert, the Prince Regent's mistress. Here in 1874 fourteen young women, twelve of them from Edinburgh, gathered to form the nucleus of the new school. It took Sophia three years to induce the Royal Free Hospital in neighbouring Gray's Inn Road to become a teaching hospital and to accept her students. Her sympathisers included Mrs Garrett Anderson, Darwin and Huxley, and thanks to their agitation in 1877 the Royal Free Hospital agreed to become associated with the London School of Medicine for Women. The Medical Register, closed to women for the past twenty years, was re-opened to them; Sophia Jex-Blake, already an MD of Berne, then became legally qualified. The Royal College of Physicians and the Royal College of Surgeons that year decided after considerable opposition to recognise the new women's medical school. Alas, at this point the British Medical Association passed a resolution it was not to revoke until 1892 to ban women from membership.

By the time Helena arrived on the scene in 1908 the women's medical school had become affiliated to the University of London. It had been enlarged and extended three times, the last in 1901. Neighbouring houses had been acquired and incorporated into a four-storeyed building round a quadrangle. The address of the London (Royal Free Hospital) School of Medicine for Women was now 8 Hunter Street. Another milestone was achieved in the year of Helena's entry and is recorded in the 1908 Annual Report of the Royal Free Hospital:

> The Council of the School are to be congratulated upon the success which has at last crowned their efforts to obtain the consent of the Royal College of Physicians and the Royal College of Surgeons to the admittance of women to all their examinations.

By 1915 the only qualifications still closed to women were the medical degrees of Oxford and Cambridge.

Helena was the 915th woman to enrol since the formation of the medical school thirty-four years earlier. Her fees for the whole five-year course were £160, and she was one of twenty-three new students that year among a total of 146 already in training in the school and hospital. As she had already taken the Preliminary Science examination at Cheltenham she went straight in to the second year, one of thirteen girls. Today the Royal Free Hospital Medical School has over five hundred students of either sex. It pleased Helena greatly before her death that her only granddaughter, Miranda Wright, was among their number. By then the Royal Free Hospital had moved to Hampstead, with nearly 900 beds compared with 165 when Helena was a student, leaving a skeleton of the medical school in Hunter Street to be eventually incorporated within the Hampstead block.

The curriculum today bears little resemblance to that provided for Helena. In her day the students spent the mornings in the laboratories or in the dissecting room and the afternoons in the library reading their textbooks. The tutorial system had not been thought of, but lectures were given by recognised university teachers. Nowadays most students do not dissect corpses; the dissections are prepared by technicians and the demonstrations are displayed for them, but Helena and her friend Peggy Martland shared a cadaver with five other pairs of students, two to each limb, two to the head and neck, and two to the chest and abdomen. One girl read aloud to her partner from Cunningham's *Manual of Anatomy*, while the other wielded the scalpel, and, having removed the skin, painstakingly laid out the nerves, arteries and veins in relation to the organs and muscles. Much more time is spent today on the science of biochemistry, which has replaced the old-style inorganic chemistry. This does not make the work any less enjoyable than Helena found it, but it brings to the student much earlier the clinical significance of the subject and reflects the sophisticated advances in modern medicine. Helena's granddaughter was not required to spend her time working on anaesthetised cats, or pithed frogs as in Helena's day and there has had to be a totally new emphasis on the actions of drugs which were not known to Helena.

She had taken up medicine quite unaware of what it would entail. Nor had she considered the possibility that she would ever need to earn her own living. She looked on the study and practice of medicine as one of the bonuses that life would provide for her, and she was not disappointed. Student life turned out to be even more rewarding than she had anticipated. She enjoyed learning the detailed anatomy of the arm of 'Joseph' as their cadaver was somewhat incongruously labelled. But Peggy wrinkled her nose. 'Smells of pheasant to me,' was all she said.

At the beginning of their first term, the new students were addressed by the Vice-Dean, a young gynaecologist, Miss (later Dame)

Louisa Aldrich-Blake, the second woman doctor to receive the DBE, who was to become one of the most distinguished surgeons of her day. As the fourth Dean she played a large part in the development of the medical school and was mainly responsible for doubling its size. Helena instantly realised that she was in the presence of 'an absolutely outstanding personality and I determined to cultivate her friendship'.

Louisa Aldrich-Blake subsequently exerted a great influence on her, and as surgeon to the Elizabeth Garrett Anderson Hospital, and later the Royal Free Hospital, helped Helena considerably in her gynaecological training—Helena kept her photograph on her desk throughout her own life and was desolated when Louisa Aldrich-Blake died.

The two women had certain characteristics in common. Louisa, born in 1865, had entered the London School of Medicine for Women in the year of Helena's birth, one of eight new students. Like Helena she came from a financially secure background, and was quite un-domesticated. When asked by her biographer, Lord Riddell, how she came to be indifferent to worldly success she replied, 'Never having been compelled to earn my living I have been freed from the strivings that inevitably beset the lives of most professional people.'[1]

She and Helena were both immune to jealousy. One of Helena's close friends believes that this freedom from the baser emotions enabled her to put into practice herself the controversial views she expressed in her books about divorce and 'infidelity'—matters which many people still find difficult to accept, or even understand.

Both Louisa Aldrich-Blake and Helena were committed to the cause of women, which they furthered with single-mindedness, but without giving any support for the suffrage movement. Both abhorred the militancy shown by some of the pioneers, including Elizabeth Garrett Anderson, who was a conspicuous figure at militant demonstrations. In 1908, the year when Helena became a medical student, Elizabeth, then aged seventy-two, had felt constrained to obey Mrs Pankhurst's call to 'Rush the House of Commons', and on 18 October joined a raid on Parliament entailing the inevitable police scuffles. Her sister Millicent Fawcett, with whom she had marched in a 13,000-strong peaceful procession, was appalled at her militant action, and before her death Elizabeth admitted to her that she had been guilty of misjudgement.

[1] *Dame Louisa Aldrich–Blake* by Lord Riddell, Hodder & Stoughton Ltd, undated.

In fact Elizabeth Garrett Anderson taught her students that, 'The first thing women must learn is to dress like ladies and behave like gentlemen,' but Louisa Aldrich-Blake believed that women should earn their place in professional life as if they *were* men, and be judged on their merits, though she objected strongly to 'mannish' women. As she said in her inaugural address to the new entrants:

> If women are going to compete with men they must be equally efficient . . . You cannot have two standards of efficiency . . . The sooner women students get that idea out of their heads, if it is there, the better. We talk too much about competing with men . . . Why think about competition? If you are good at your work you are certain to succeed and if you are not you are certain to fail.

The world in which Helena found herself at the School of Medicine was predominantly composed of women. Her fellow students were all girls, and with the exception of the Professor of Anatomy for a short time, she was taught by women heads of departments and women demonstrators. Tom Hill remained her only friend of the opposite sex. Inevitably romantic friendships developed among this closely-knit feminine community. Helena's ties with Peggy Martland began when they were students, and lasted throughout their lives. On 3 September 1913 Peggy wrote during a train journey 'Somewhere in Somerset':

> Helena darling
>
> I found I couldn't wait any longer, and as soon as the train showed the faintest sign of stopping anywhere I stuck out my head and roared for notepaper with such insistence that I got it—of sorts. I'm still feeling torn most painfully in two, with the bigger bit left behind . . . Oh, you witch can you half guess how you have transfixed the whole of my life for me? Just think! I've known you four whole years more or less and only just begun to love you properly. And it wouldn't have happened even now if you hadn't ever so quietly, pulled and shoved and kicked and worried, and held me by the scruff of my neck while you loved me into life. I *am* a most colossal ass! Why you took the trouble in the beginning is more than I can imagine . . . I love you and love you, darling friend of mine . . . Thank you for everything and bless you always.
>
> Peggy

Their friendship continued after Helena's marriage. When the Wrights had left for China, Peggy, who never married, wrote:

Helena Beloved

Life is just a dazed hurt which seems to get worse instead of better as I begin to realise that you won't all come bundling back to 49 Cumberland Place in a week or two. The last week has been a nightmare in which I somehow could only go stolidly on in a lumpish way saying none of the things I badly wanted to say. Thank heaven we understand one another without getting things said.

Beloved, are you getting in orgies of sleep to make up at least a bit? You need to. It's a relief to think these last horrible days are over for you. Nothing else can be so bad, can it? . . . Darling heart. I want to take you in my arms and kiss peace into your tired self. My love goes with you all the time.

Much love, to the Peter boy and a kiss to the babies.

Darling, I love you.

Peggy
31A Mortimer Street, W1, 23.11.21

Helena became a member of the London Inter-Faculty Christian Union and of the Student Christian Movement, both of which had active branches within the medical school. Rena Carswell, whom Helena had met in 1906, was now the SCM secretary for women's colleges and later the secretary for all the university branches. She and Helena used to attend the SCM summer conferences, at one of which Helena met the famous 'Billy' Temple, already a bishop, and his mother. According to Helena they were 'a devoted couple'.

In 1913 Helena was put on the Executive by the English head-quarters of the Student Christian Movement, an interdenominational active organisation, and in the same year was a delegate to the World Student Christian Federation meeting at Lake Mohawk in the USA. The President was John R. Mott, then leader of the World Student Christian Movement, who had earlier made a deep impression on Helena when speaking at the Albert Hall in 1910, and had so moved

---

Long summer holidays at Chrzanow with Polish and German cousins. Rosa Lowenfeld (seated) with all her sons, their wives and children. Helena, the eldest grandchild, is beside her grandmother, with her mother's hand resting on her shoulder, and her father is in the foreground with his daughter Margaret astride.

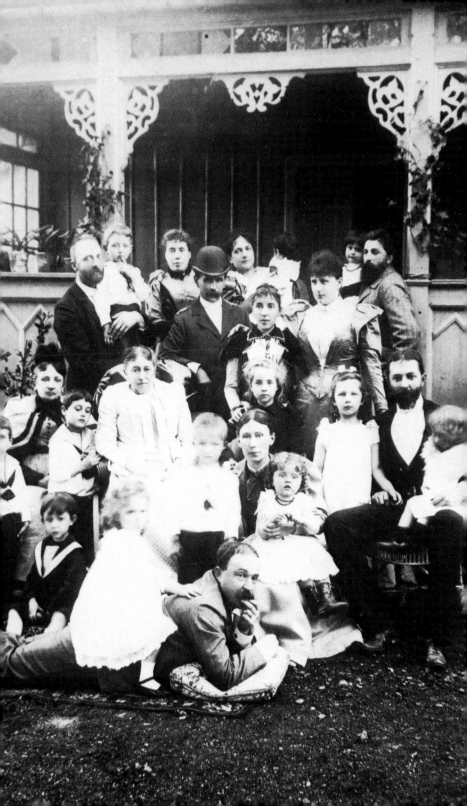

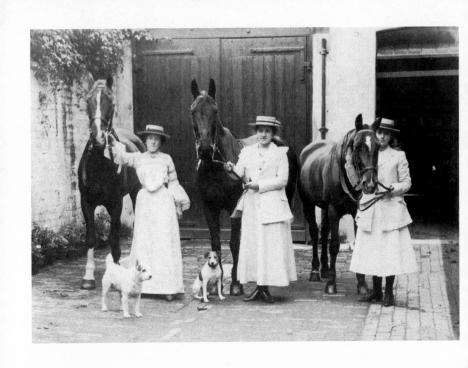

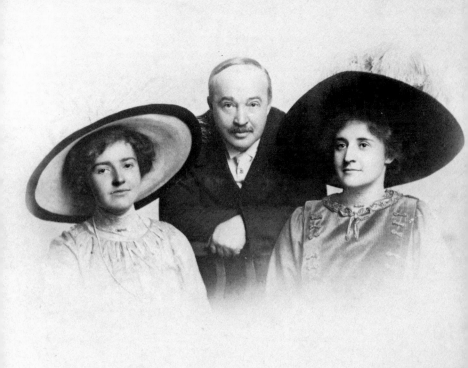

her that she thereupon signed a Student Volunteer card committing herself to work in the mission field. This led later to her active period of medical work in China.

Meanwhile she was happy and fulfilled all day at the London School of Medicine, but utterly miserable in her mother's house at Hounslow. She and Margaret found Frank Quicke increasingly intolerable. The year in which Margaret had promised her mother she would not see her father was up, and both girls were now in regular contact with Henry Lowenfeld. Recognising the roots of their unhappiness, he came to the rescue for the second time, not as at Little Brickhill with a temporary solution, but with a more lasting arrangement.

Alice seems hardly to have been consulted, but in January 1910 he took over the lease of 49 Great Cumberland Place. It was a large five-storeyed house near Marble Arch and Henry engaged as chatelaine Lady Alice Leslie, an aristocrat, eighteenth in line to the throne, who was then about sixty. The girls loved her, christened her 'Dobbin' and got on with their own lives in which she never interfered. Helena bicycled every day to the School of Medicine while Lady Alice ran the house and managed the servants. She brought her own maid and found a French one for the girls. She answered the telephone amiably when their mother telephoned, as she did daily. Visits to Hounslow had become painless because they were strictly limited. Alice Quicke would send her carriage for the girls and she herself came frequently to see them when Henry was not expected. There was peace at last. Henry was welcomed whenever he chose to call. By now he had put in extra bathrooms and a Steinway grand piano, while Lady Alice created an environment in which both the girls could comfortably pursue their medical training. She expected only the mildest customary conventions to be observed, but she and both girls automatically dressed for dinner every night. As Helena later observed, 'Dobbin could not have eaten her dinner unless she had changed and was waited on by a parlour maid.'

One evening when Helena returned home she found Henry

(above) *Cheltenham schooldays. Helena (centre), with her mother (left) and sister (right), grew up hating horses and dressing up.*

(left) *Father and daughters, Margaret (left) and Helena (right). Henry Lowenfeld was probably the strongest influence on Helena's life. As he wrote to her: 'Are you not my child in every sense of the word? . . . Everything that is sacred to you is sacred to me . . . working with life and soul I have never failed in anything.'*

Lowenfeld at tea. On her plate lay a necklace. 'Lest you should think those are my idea of good beads, Helena,' he said, 'I may tell you they are nothing to the quality of pearls I shall give you when you take your final examinations—and fail them.' Father and daughter looked at one another. 'The bribe is not enough,' said Helena. It was his last and only attempt to dissuade her from following her chosen path, but first he asked her to do one thing for him. He would agree to her being a doctor, but he wanted her first to understand what she would be sacrificing. Would she, to please him, first do the London Season? They struck a bargain. She would do as he wished and if at the end of the year the conventional social life failed to satisfy her she would return to her medical studies. She saw now why Papa had installed Lady Alice.

Having once given her father her word, Helena brought to the Season all her native wit and interest. For some reason she disapproved of the theatre, but she did everything else demanded of her, lunches, dinners, and balls. Though she groaned inwardly she, who hated dressing up, went shopping with Lady Alice for dresses, shoes, hats and gloves. At midday they would be at home unless at a lunch party. After lunch they had an hour's rest before sallying forth with visiting cards and a taxi-whistle at the ready. If by good luck the hostess was out the cards would be left with one corner turned down. Evenings found Helena in a dress two inches above the instep, stockings of the same colour and satin shoes dyed to match.

As well as falling in with Lady Alice's plans Helena would add suggestions of her own. When they gave a dinner party she went out into the country in search of wild cherry for the table vases instead of the conventional roses and carnations. When it was their turn to give a dance she had the staircases and landings hung with a green screen of smilax which wafted in the breeze. She persuaded the florist to decorate the ballroom ceiling with yellow and purple irises fixed with their heads pointing downwards. But it was all in vain. At the end of the summer she had not found a prospective husband, or indeed even one interesting young man. 'Can't you like *any* of them?' Lady Alice had asked despairingly. Apparently not. Henry admitted defeat. 'Well, girls, you've won,' he told his daughters, and Helena was free to go back to medicine.

It had not been a totally fruitless exercise. Both Helena and her father had learnt to know one another better and their early love for each other had been renewed. Helena had always found her father interesting. Now she watched the way in which he managed his business, and they would go for drives together. Once on such an excursion he noticed there were flag sellers on the street but was not impressed with their performance. What could they sell instead of flags? Roses for the blind, made by the blind. And so was born Queen Alexandra's Rose Day. Henry introduced an organiser. Margaret and her cousin Rösel Lowenfeld with society girls in white sold the roses which were designed at the Royal School of Needlework. The prettiest girls were photographed with the Lord Mayor and Lady Mayoress. Queen Alexandra was interviewed and bestowed her patronage. It was all a great success, and typical of Henry that he remained in the background himself taking no credit. Increasingly occupied with his business affairs, he was now buying estates in South America, and was concerned with the Investment Registry Ltd., as the Universal Stock Exchange Ltd. was now called, dealing with world investment policy. He had moved his capital to France and in 1912 settled with Frania in an opulent apartment in Paris in the avenue du Bois de Boulogne. Here both girls could conveniently visit him at weekends by the Golden Arrow.

Henry had accepted his failure over his daughter Helena's excursion into the social life of fashionable London. It had been for her only an amusing interlude, after which she thankfully returned to student life, bicycling every day to hospital. She passed the Intermediate Medical examination in 1912, having had to re-take the pharmacology examination. Being on her own admission 'of a lazy nature', she had not exerted herself unduly over pharmacology which she said was just a matter of memory. She had found that 'the intelligence of examiners never seems overwhelming'.

The next years were spent in clinical training on the wards. She had often walked through to the Gray's Inn Road from the medical school along Handel Street into the beautiful St George's Burial Ground where Oliver Cromwell's granddaughter Jane, who died in 1726, lies in a tomb she shares with her husband Thomas Gibson, M D, physician general of the Army, as the inscription notes. He died in London 1722, aged seventy-seven years. Helena must have sat by the grave on sunny days among the old worn tombstones with her friends during breaks, as countless students have done since. The far end of the garden, beyond the Braille Herb Garden, leads into the Gray's Inn Road, almost opposite the stone entrance arch of the old hospital that opened into the front square with its four great plane trees. It was known as the Quad, and there the 'honoraries' would park their Rolls-Royces. The wards were on either side with operating theatres on the top floor on the left. The Out Patient Department and laboratories were reached through a passage, always known as 'the duodenum' on account of its shape.

The 'honoraries' were aptly named, for in those days their services were unpaid. These consultants taught students who, as future general practitioners, would refer patients to them at their 'rooms' in Harley or Wimpole Streets, an area known colloquially as 'The Devil's Acre'. Their private practice constituted their main source of income in return for the supervision of their hospital patients' treatment. When Helena was a student there were no private wards at the Royal Free Hospital and private cases were treated in nursing homes. The 'voluntary' hospitals were supported by public contributions and all were permanently in debt, running to as much as £200,000. They were administered by a lay committee chaired by a public figure. A fleet of almoners, the forerunners of today's social workers, were occupied in determining the amount of money, if any, each patient could contribute towards the cost of hospital care.

A new experience was in store for Helena. She was in future to be taught by men, and the only woman honorary she remembered among the galaxy of new teachers was Mary Scharlieb, consulting physician for Diseases of Women who was also consulting surgeon to the New Hospital for Women, later renamed in 1917 the Elizabeth Garrett Anderson Hospital. The other leading lights among the honoraries were the surgeons Joseph Cunning and James Berry. Berry (later Sir James) was Helena's favourite. He had a club foot and an imperfectly repaired harelip. The resulting speech defect partially obscured his comments, especially when in the operating theatre he was wearing a mask. His wife Frances was his anaesthetist, and no mask could obscure the arguments which passed between them. 'Give her more,' would be countered by 'That's my job. She's had plenty.' The atmosphere in the theatre, according to Helena, was 'anything but formal'. James Berry was a quick operator who specialised in goitres and cleft palates. The day had not dawned when a tube is passed down the windpipe and the amount of anaesthetic controlled at a distance by the anaesthetist. Husband and wife had frequently to share the head of the patient for operations when the anaesthetic required a mask over the face. Helene noticed that marital bickering never interfered with good theatre discipline and she believed that surgeon and anaesthetist were really in fundamental accord with one another.

During their hospital training students spent three months in each of the special departments during which they worked, in Helena's phrase, at 'playing the doctor'. They were allocated a number of patients and were responsible for keeping the notes under the supervision of the house officer, and had to produce these on the day of the honorary's weekly 'round'. On the great day the 'chief' would be accompanied by his house surgeon or house physician, as the case might be. Then came Sister, followed at a respectful distance by Staff Nurse, at least two other nurses, appropriately starched, and then the students wearing in Helena's time the regulation brown holland overall—only 'proper' doctors rated a white coat. Scrupulous ward preparation had been made. All patients would be lying in bed, their clean unruffled sheets turned down with military precision. Any crying child would be relegated to the sluice room for the duration of the round. No one spoke unless addressed directly by the great man. The procession divided round each bed so that Sister stood opposite the chief at the head of the bed, while he read the notes, examined the patient and questioned the students about diagnosis and treatment.

The authority of Sister on the ward was paramount, not only over her nurses, but also the students. Helena's first three months were spent on the medical side. On her first day Sister told her which patients had been allocated to her, including a 'heart' case. She had no idea how to deal with any of them, but, undaunted, she set off to talk to the latter and returned to Sister with the information that the 'heart' lady's legs were swollen so it must be a 'leg' case. 'I think you'll find the two are not incompatible, Miss Lowenfeld,' said Sister. Next time she was baffled she went to the house physician for help, and asked him what she was supposed to hear down her stethoscope, to which the young man airily replied, 'Oh, a few bubbles and squeaks.' This she duly inscribed in the notes, only to learn when the day of the ward round dawned that she should have described the sounds she was supposed to hear as 'râles' (from the French râler, to rattle) and 'rhonchi' (from the Greek rhonchos, to snore). No matter, Miss Lowenfeld was not easily crushed, and told the honorary that bubbles and squeaks was what the house physician called them. The incident left her with a poor opinion of male house physicians.

The Children's Ward was filled with acutely ill children suffering from both medical and surgical conditions. Chorea and rickets were common complaints in those days. Chorea, which we never see now, caused uncoordinated movements often followed by permanent heart damage due to acute rheumatism. This common and distressing condition vanished from the scene when rheumatic fever declined at the end of the Thirties after the sulphonamide drugs became available in 1937 and were used in the treatment of streptococcal infections, but in Helena's student days there was no effective treatment for chorea.

On the other hand rickets was then curable in hospital if cod liver oil was given. The dietary cause of the disease was previously unrecognised and no one understood that vitamin deficiency affected the bones. Rickets was prevalent among the poorly-fed children whom Helena encountered on the ward, and only disappeared once the role of Vitamin D was established, and babies were given cod liver oil.

The main surgical condition which Helena saw on the Children's Ward has also vanished; tuberculosis of bones, causing suppurating ulcers that required frequent dressings, and often surgery, was common in her day. Tuberculous bone infections differed from pulmonary tuberculosis, and were due to drinking raw milk from cattle infected with the bovine type of tuberculosis before the days of pasteurisation. The testing of herds and eradication of infected animals has eliminated a condition for which James Berry was often required to operate. Antibiotics were unknown; ear, nose and throat infections were rife, and could lead to infections of the mastoid, for which there was only surgical treatment. Helena recalled that if the tonsils were at all enlarged this was an indication for their removal, so that 'Ts and As' figured frequently on Mr Gay French's operating list.

Helena was especially happy during her three months in the Casualty Department, which suited her temperament. She liked dealing with people and their immediate problems. No two days were alike and she found emergencies more absorbing than a regular assignment. Students had to assess each new case, but could call on the junior resident doctor if necessary. In this the student would be guided by the Casualty Sister with her years of experience. Helena could deal herself with children who had pushed beads up their nostrils or down their ears in the boredom engendered by lack of toys. It was the era of black fogs and there would be smuts to take out of eyes. Toothache was a recurring problem.

Then there were the chronic conditions, such as neglected varicose ulcers in both men and women, necessitating regular dressings over many weeks. The word 'sore' was as vague then as today. Impetigo resulted from scratching the skin and infection. But Helena preferred all this to non-clinical subjects such as Public Health when students learnt about drains, water supplies, slaughter-houses, and crematoria, not realising that preventive medicine would eliminate in years to come much chronic illness.

Mental illness was covered in a single visit by all the students in Helena's year to the asylum at Bedlam. Each girl could meet one case. Helena's was a man who told her he was made of glass. For the first time she encountered someone whose link with reality no longer existed, and with whom there was no means of communication. For him medicine offered only physical protection from his own tragic and melancholy state, sleeping draughts and aperients. Treatment of mental states lay many years ahead, there was no teaching whatever about psychology, and the sexual problems Helena was to encounter twenty years later were either unrecognised or unmentionable.

She had two particularly happy periods in her training, both connected with women patients. Babies were not delivered in hospital and mothers were only admitted in an emergency; they were attended in their homes by students who had never seen them before. The students lived in a house in Mecklenburgh Square during their month 'on the district' which extended north as far as the Pentonville Road. Each girl, on a rota, conducted twenty cases. When the prospective father knocked on the door the 'doctor' would sally forth with him into the unknown, while he carried her bag. On arrival she would find an amateur midwife or 'gamp' in attendance to provide hot water and reassurance, and the woman's bed would be protected with layers of brown paper. There the embryo doctor had to sit patiently while the gamp might gossip and bugs fall from the ceiling. If things went wrong the student could send the father back to base with a 'pink' asking for help. A 'pink' was only a slip of pink paper, but legend had it that the system was an extension of the days when the message slip had been dipped in blood. There was a tale, no doubt apocryphal, of the student who wrote on her 'pink', 'Baby dead, mother collapsed. Not feeling too well myself.'

The Royal Free district abutted on to that covered by the young gentlemen from St Bartholomew's Hospital, so some patients were looked after by Royal Free students while their neighbours came into the Bart's orbit. These men students had the reputation, according to Helena's information, of being 'very careless with the afterbirth'. She supposed this meant that the Royal Free girls were better at tidying up before they left at the end of the job. Though she found it enjoyable, it was a time of intense activity and responsibility, and to ease the strain she began to smoke cigarettes.

The other period of happiness was while she was a temporary student at the New Hospital for Women. Royal Free students could do an elective period at one of the two women's hospitals, the other being the South London on Clapham Common. Helena jumped at the chance of the former hospital because there she could sit at the feet of her heroine Louisa Aldrich–Blake, attend her out-patient clinics, and watch her operate. She went on her rounds in the wards, and compared her favourably with the men surgeons at the Royal Free.

Suddenly the tempo of her life changed. That summer Helena and Margaret were due to join their father at Bayreuth for the festival. On 27 July 1914 Henry wrote from Marienbad, where he was taking one of his regular cures, that they must arrive on 3 August to be in time for *Parsifal* on the fourth. Applying to Cook's for their tickets, Helena learnt that none were being issued beyond the Dutch frontier. No reason was given and Helena was mystified. Had she bought their tickets and travelled a few days earlier she and her sister might have been caught on the Continent for the duration of the First World War, declared on 4 August. Henry Lowenfeld returned to his native Austrian Poland where he was to base himself for the next four years, and Helena did not see him until the following year when they met in neutral Switzerland.

Henry did not waste the war years when he was debarred from returning to Paris, and moved between Chrzanow, Cracow and Vienna. He became the leader of the Society for the Foundation of Polish Legions and in Cracow he set up 'Zalal' (Society to Help the People). Under his direction Zalal bought, mainly from Russia, clothing and war-time food such as sugar and jam in short supply, which was sold to the rich at thirty per cent below market price and to the poor at a hundred per cent below this figure. Zalal proved so successful that out of its profits it was able to extend the boarding section of the high school in Cracow and establish bursaries.

Meanwhile, Henry was also building up for himself a major antiques collection in Vienna. He had the ear of those who were influential and discovered that the art treasures of the murdered heir to the Austrian throne were to be auctioned privately. To avoid possible embarrassment over the way these antiques had been acquired, the professional art dealers were not invited to attend the auction, but Henry went. He had wired instructions to Adolf to mortgage the whole of his Chrzanow property and gave him power of attorney. As Adolf has described in his unpublished memoir, *Seventy-Six Years of Chrzanow*, a wagon-load of enormously valuable antiques duly arrived at Chrzanow and were stored in the Billiard House until Henry went there in 1921. He then set up a huge exhibition to which he invited the leading art experts, including the Director of the Cracow Museum, before despatching the best pieces to his Paris apartment.

[6]

The First World War

On 14 October 1914 while Helena was working in London she got a wire from her father, 'Manage all my businesses'. Henry gave her control of his account at the Haymarket branch of the Westminster Bank, where his balance stood at £11,000, and instructed her to get a second mortgage on the Apollo Theatre. From the manager of the theatre she received a weekly rent of £200, and on this she had to look after three of her father's ex-mistresses, and pay Lady Alice's house-keeping expenses at 49 Great Cumberland Place, as well as her own and Margaret's out-of-pocket expenses. She took all this in her stride, admitting that she was incapable of worrying about money and 'quite easy to cheat'. Lady Alice could only suggest two economies: they could, she thought, forgo the services of the man who came daily to wash the palms, and dispense with the weekly visit of the clock winder.

Helena accepted the control of the Apollo Theatre, where the following sign appeared in due course, 'Dr Helena Lowenfeld is hereby entitled to sell Beer, Wines, Spirits and Cigarettes on these premises'. By then she was qualified as a doctor, but earlier than she had envisaged. Shortly after the outbreak of war the Conjoint Board of the Royal Colleges of Physicians and Surgeons introduced a modified qualifying examination in order that women, by taking this examina-tion, could fill the places of men who were needed in the armed forces. Helena failed this examination on her first attempt. Full of her usual confidence she had gone to the examination hall in Queen Square for the oral examination, having already sat the papers. She was never one to take anything uncritically, and having disagreed with a particular treatment favoured by the examiner in Gynaecology, she told him so. She then offered the examiner in Medicine the gratuitous information that she considered the question he had just asked her 'rather a silly one'. She later admitted she had been misguided, although she held to her opinions, which cost her her failure. Before she re-sat the Conjoint

Examination she wrote to the secretary of the Board asking if she could be examined by other examiners than those who had failed her. Three months later she passed successfully.

The following year, in 1915, she took the University of London degree of MB, BS without difficulty. The examination was remarkable from her point of view in constituting a milestone in her development of extra-sensory perception, in which she was already interested. In the Pathology viva the examiner had handed her a museum specimen to identify. 'Actinomycosis of the liver,' she replied unhesitatingly. The examiner was duly impressed, smiled from ear to ear, and told her no other candidate had recognised the condition. She did not tell him that she had never heard of actinomycosis, let alone seen an example of it in the human liver. The words surprised her as she uttered what turned out to be the correct diagnosis. It was her first experience of what she believed to be telepathy, whereby she was able to communicate with the brain of a total stranger.

Within a year of the declaration of war Helena and her friend Peggy Martland were working as the first resident women doctors in the Out Patient Department in Camden Town of the Hampstead General Hospital. Any cases they could not treat themselves they referred to the main hospital for admittance. The job was unpaid, but Helena and Peggy earned three guineas for attendance at the mortuary whenever a post mortem examination on a coroner's case was made. A victim of a fatal accident was known as a BID (Brought in Dead), and Helena recalled that on three successive Fridays a BID was brought in at exactly 5 o'clock from an accident on the neighbouring railway bridge. Both the newly qualified young doctors appear to have given satisfaction, and at the end of six months they were transferred to the main hospital at the top of Haverstock Hill where Peggy Martland became the house physician, and Helena the house surgeon. As such she found herself responsible to six honorary surgeons each of whom differed in their post-operative care of patients. One, she later remembered, required all his patients to have only ginger ale for a week after the operation.

It was all good experience, but unfortunately it did not last. Her Germanic name had already aroused suspicion while Helena was still a student. Soon after the outbreak of war a policeman had appeared at their home in Great Cumberland Place asking where she had been born and saying she had been named as a spy. Helena was glad to tell him she had been born in Brixton if he cared to see her passport, and was the daughter of a 'friendly alien'. She had also been aware of spy mania during the M B examination when she had again been asked to produce her passport. After three months in her job at the Hampstead General Hospital, in May 1915, she received a letter from the Chairman of the Lay Board:

> Dear Dr Lowenfeld,
> We have reason to believe your continued presence in the hospital is not to the hospital's advantage. We therefore ask you to resign your present post . . .

Helena was enraged but had no alternative but to comply with the wishes of the Board, and Peggy Martland resigned in protest at the injustice meted out to her friend. Helena and Margaret then spent the next few weeks in Lucerne with their father.

Returning to England, Helena answered an advertisement for a house surgeon at the Hospital for Sick Children, Great Ormond Street, and was accepted. She was the only girl on the staff and found herself in a predominantly male environment. She could not understand how the young doctors could put up with their bleak surroundings and set about improving the residents' quarters. She would go out early in the morning on her bicycle to Covent Garden market, where she persuaded altruistic sellers to give her flowers 'for the Children's Hospital'. All her life Helena was to love flowers and enjoy arranging them, and she filled the hospital Common Room with vases, which, apart from a young Canadian doctor, no one else seemed to appreciate.

It was for her a period of great professional satisfaction. She worked for the famous surgeon of the day, Arbuthnot Lane, with whom she developed a happy relationship. He had already given his name to certain surgical instruments and an operation which he had devised for the repair of cleft palate, which differed from that favoured by James Berry. Arbuthnot Lane would look over the top of his mask when Helena was assisting him in the theatre and say with a smile, 'I know you come from the opposite party, Miss Lowenfeld, but please note how this repair should be effected.' During one of these sessions a message was brought in for Dr Lowenfeld from the manager of the Apollo Theatre, Mr Tom B. Davies, who wanted to know if he could order new seats for the stalls. Helena sent back a message saying not the stalls, but he could get new seats for the dress circle, which apparently amused Arbuthnot Lane.

This period in Arbuthnot Lane's career coincided with the

development of his irrational conviction that the bowel contents could poison the system, by a process which he called 'auto-intoxication'. He believed this to be curable only by the removal of the whole bowel, and Helena was sometimes required to assist him in this serious and potentially fatal operation—a formidable treatment for a non-existent condition. Lane later ceased to treat 'auto-intoxication' surgically, and relied instead on enormous doses of liquid paraffin. Once when he was asked to examine in surgery in Manchester, he arrived with a large bottle of liquid paraffin as a gift for his hostess, the wife of the professor of surgery.

At the end of this job Helena and Arbuthnot Lane parted with mutual regret. She was used to male society by now and had refused two offers of marriage. In 1913 she had been briefly engaged to Jim Wallace, a Canadian student she had met at the World Federation Student Christian Conference at Lake Mohawk in the USA. He had come to England afterwards, and she had taken him over to Paris, accompanied by Lady Alice Leslie, to meet her father. She broke the engagement after a fortnight, and Jim went off to Moscow. His brother Bill turned up on a week's leave from the trenches in France while Helena was at Great Ormond Street. They spent her time off duty together, and she took a day off to show him the English countryside, which Arbuthnot Lane told her was 'very sensible' of her.

Once Helena had completed her three training posts and left the Hospital for Sick Children she looked about her for a job which would directly help the war effort. She was a fervent pacifist, and has said that if she had been a man she would have been a conscientious objector. She would not join the uniformed services, but wanted to work in a military hospital. A group of Scottish women doctors had formed a unit in 1914 which they offered to the War Office. The offer was declined, but the French Red Cross was glad to have the ladies, who began to work together in several French centres. A group, which included Louisa Garrett Anderson, Elizabeth's daughter, opened a hospital in Claridge's Hotel in Paris, which so impressed Lord Esher on a visit of inspection that he pointed out the folly of allowing women doctors to leave England.

Ferreting up and down the corridors of Whitehall, Helena discovered from the War Office that she could work under a Colonel Hurry Fenwick as a civilian junior surgeon at the Bethnal Green Hospital, a large municipal hospital which the Army Medical Services had taken over for military casualties. It suited her admirably as the Number 6 bus from Marble Arch put her down daily outside the hospital. She was in charge of Mercy Ward, and again found herself in another all-male environment, but here she was the only doctor not in the RAMC. She worked on a rota with a New Zealand surgeon, a veteran of the Boer War, called Colonel Fell. According to Helena he was rosy-cheeked, with a white moustache and looked like Father Christmas. This happy pair formed themselves into a team, working as surgeon and anaesthetist and reversing their roles to add variety.

The war itself seems barely to have impinged on their life. There was the odd Zeppelin raid, and one night all the lights in the hospital failed while Helena was trying to control a severe haemorrhage, but she continued to work by torchlight. Otherwise this period was apparently medically uneventful. But one day late in July 1916 Helena saw walking down a corridor towards her a tall, thin and, as she described him, 'strikingly good-looking' young man in uniform. He turned out to be an RAMC officer on sick leave from a casualty clearing station in France, who had been posted to Bethnal Green for light duties. The young man, a Captain H. W. S. Wright, joined the Lowenfeld-Fell team, turning the partnership into a trio. The three worked harmoniously and with the same interchange of roles as Helena and Colonel Fell, except that whoever was doing the surgery now had an assistant. To Helena the young Captain Wright, five years her junior, appeared as 'a rock, signifying strength and gentleness', and the relationship deepened.

Helena did not care for his first name, which was Henry, perhaps because that was her father's name, but she rationalised her prejudice by saying that the footmen at Lowndes Square had always been addressed as 'Henry'. 'You're Peter,' she soon told their new recruit, and 'Peter' he remained for the rest of his life. When in due course Peter broached the subject of marriage Helena became alarmed and asked him if his ideas of liberty would be as wide as hers. Marriage looked ominously like a cage, and if there was one thing Helena was determined about it was that she would not be caged. Moreover, what she had seen of her parents' marriage was not encouraging, and her mother's second marriage was an even greater disaster. 'I like you, but I don't like the thought of marriage,' she told Peter as they went home on the Number 6 bus together after a heavy day in the operating theatre. He did not mention the subject again for six months.

At the end of this period, in return for his forbearance and what

Helena described as his 'endless generosity', Helena proposed in March 1917 that they should have a trial engagement, so that each could meet the other's family, and if it worked they would go ahead with marriage, provided Peter realised that her work was more important than anything else including him, and that she would not give it up on any account. She was wary of an emotional relationship, and considered passion far too risky to contemplate. She based her hopes for their marriage on similarity of interests, solid respect and pleasure in the other's company, which left proximity and affection as the basis for a physical relationship which became 'as natural as stroking a cat'.

The balance was tilted in Peter's favour when she discovered, wonder of wonders, that he too had been a Student Volunteer, was a Christian like herself, and intended to go to China as a missionary. She took him off to Liberty's to buy an engagement ring, choosing her favourite stone, an opal. If Tom Hill had had any expectations of marriage to Helena they were now doomed, and the emerald pendant he gave Helena as a wedding present became known in the family as 'Tom's tear'.

Before their marriage Helena took Peter to Geneva where Henry was staying in a hotel with Frania. Helena had not seen her step-mother since the early meeting at Chrzanow when Frania had so upset Alice by her appearance on the scene. Henry Lowenfeld was still exactly as Helena had last seen him, sitting with one leg under the other meticulously cutting sheets of black tissue paper with his nail scissors into pictures and patterns he fixed to a white background. He appeared oblivious to Frania's obvious discontent. Henry Lowenfeld had the ability, which his daughter Helena inherited, to detach his mind completely from a situation he did not choose to notice. Frania had taken exception to the presence in another hotel in the town of a young Polish school teacher, Mieczslawa Hülle Gadomska, known in the family as Gnaus, or as 'The Serpent', and sometimes 'The Black One'. Miss Gadomska had been Henry's constant companion after his return to Chrzanow at the outset of the war, and it had been alleged in the family—and fiercely denied by Helena—that Henry used his daughter Margaret's passport to effect Miss Gadomska's entry into Switzerland.

Helena found herself sympathetic towards Frania, but this did not prevent her, when Frania asked her to persuade Henry to get rid of Miss Gadomska, from pointing out that here was simply an example of history repeating itself. Instead of obliging Frania, Henry set up Miss Gadomska, thirty-five years his junior, in a small cosmetic business in France. She remained with him and looked after him until his death in a Paris hotel in 1931 while Frania returned to Warsaw. According to members of the Lowenfeld family who knew her at Chrzanow 'this simple modest woman' did not deserve the epithets 'Serpent' or 'Black One'.

After seeing her father Helena went back to work at Bethnal Green Hospital, and Peter to his casualty clearing station in France in due course, only to find that he was not yet fit for duty. He was then returned to a military hospital in England, this time as a patient himself, and was later invalided out of the army. Meanwhile, Alice was delighted that Helena was to be married and set her daughter up with a conventional trousseau. She was rewarded and gratified at Robinson and Cleaver in Bond Street, where they went to buy the linen, to be served by an assistant who recognised her and remembered her address from the Lowndes Square days.

The wedding took place on 17 August 1917, at the Chapel of the Savoy. Helena wore a dress of cream satin made by the Bond Street dressmakers who had made her Court dress. Peter, on forty-eight hours' leave from his hospital, wore uniform, and so did his brother James, a dentist, who was best man. Helena could never remember who gave her away—possibly it was the hated Frank Quicke—but it was not her father, who could not come to England to see his daughter married. Margaret Lowenfeld and Peter's sister Connie were bridesmaids. There was a small family reception, after which Helena and Peter spent their two-day honeymoon in a hotel at Petworth where it rained the whole weekend and then duly returned to Great Cumberland Place.

Helena told me that neither she nor Peter had had any sexual experience until then. She was later to urge students and others to experiment before marriage, saying that 'marriage between virgins is doomed to failure'. But when I asked her if she wished she and Peter had acted other than as they did, she replied, 'I don't think so. I'm an extrovert. It's all come out properly according to my pattern. I accepted what was happening to me and did my best with it.'

That autumn Peter was transferred to a military job at Woodbridge in Suffolk where they lived temporarily in lodgings. Without contraceptives—they later relied on spermicides—Helena conceived within a month. She had to give up her work at Bethnal Green, and found pregnancy boring. In order to relieve the tedium, she took up the study of astrology and soon became convinced of the influence of the stars on human affairs. She had found a professional teacher, a Mr Kymera, who showed her how to set up a horoscope. She sent him the dates of the important events in her life, and he sent her the maps and ephemerides or astronomical tables, produced yearly at Greenwich. She could then work out the influences of the angular relationship of the planets at the time of birth to each other, and find where they were placed in the general plan of the map. This map constituted a circle divided into twelve spaces known as 'houses', each of which exerted a particular astrological influence. In each of the twelve 'houses' a planet would be in a different position and this provided her with mathematical data which she could use to calculate the expected effect. Considering that when she was over ninety she was studying how a computer worked, the astrological calculations she was working on sixty years earlier were not unduly difficult.

She was pleased to find that she and Peter were in each other's maps. Her 'house' was the House of Friends and Companions, and when Mr Kymera heard this he told Helena, 'People will be with you all your life.' No one who knew her could fail to recognise the truth of this forecast. Throughout her long life Helena was seldom alone, and her house overflowed with those who came for help or advice, or simply to see their old friend. Fundamentally she was a rescuer and few people, even strangers, called on her in vain.

Once she had learnt the rudiments of setting up a horoscope, Helena felt she had to prove the validity of her new experiment. She pressed Peter into collaboration, and together they extended their study to the other people living in their lodging house, most of whom were total strangers. Helena felt satisfied when one couple, when told the findings, insisted that the Wrights must have known facts about them of which they could not have been aware if they had not had inside information or met the couple previously. This strengthened Helena's conviction and she further proved to her own satisfaction the reliability of her astrological calculations by reference to the birth dates of members of her own family.

She was noticeably successful in casting her father's horoscope which indicated a forceful character and enormous enterprise resulting in financial success in foreign countries. Here was a man with the wish to command rather than lead, who preferred to work with his brains rather than his body. There would be more than one marriage, ill harmony in his domestic life, disappointment and quarrels. He would have two daughters, possibly clever and possibly doctors. There would be a tendency to heart trouble (which eventually caused his death) and to digestive disturbances (from which he certainly suffered).

> To sum up, this horoscope shows the native has a very superior intellect in a practical way, if less developed in a cultural or bookish sense . . .
> Victor Hugo says man is the tadpole of an angel. This tadpole seems promising because full of energy.
> HENRY LOWENFELD. Born 2.53 a.m., 1 September 1859

Meanwhile Helena's first pregnancy came to an end when the Wrights' eldest son was born on 17 June 1918. He was delivered at 49 Great Cumberland Place by a Dr Doherty. As before Helena had insisted on a woman doctor looking after her. However, Peter gave the anaesthetic, and stood up well to Helena's criticism after the event that she had expected the doctor to bring her a girl. Rena Carswell's sister took on the job of monthly nurse, and Henry Lowenfeld wired from Chrzanow, 'Greetings Henry'. The boy, destined to become a distinguished doctor, was christened Henry Beric at St James's Church, Piccadilly, but was known as 'Beric' throughout his life.

After Peter had been invalided out of the army in 1918 he was told to take six months' sick leave. He and Helena went down to Cornwall to the Land's End Hotel which was run by Tom Hill's brother, taking with them their baby Beric. It was here that a meeting of far-reaching importance took place although Helena was unaware of its significance at the time, and might not have acknowledged its importance later. By a strange coincidence Marie Stopes was staying at the same hotel on her second honeymoon. At the age of thirty-seven she had married Humphrey Roe, a rich young engineer who was to help finance the first birth control clinic in Britain on which her heart was set. It was probably the happiest time of her tortured life. Helena remembered Marie in 1918 as a graceful attractive woman sitting on the rocks in a long white lace dress. Together they would walk down to swim at Sennen Cove taking with them the baby which Helena was breast feeding.

Helena found Marie a complex character. She was the child of repressive parents who, like her own, had quarrelled constantly. She would have liked children of her own but refused her first two offers of marriage when the suitors admitted they had kissed other women. She wanted to marry a Japanese professor of botany whom she met in England, and she followed him to Japan. There she instructed him how to kiss her, a process foreign to his cultural background and, in the event, as she told the poor man, she found the experience 'quite horrid'. The blow to Marie's pride when his ardour cooled had a lasting effect on her self-esteem. Eventually in America she met Dr Reginald Ruggles Gates, a Canadian botanist, whom she married within a few weeks. She was cleverer than Dr Gates and more dominating, factors which doubtless both contributed to his impotence. Marie's innocence—or ignorance—was such that it took her three years to realise its existence, and when she divorced him at the age of thirty-six, she was still a virgin. Finding Canadian solicitors unhelpful on her terms, as was her own doctor in London and her London solicitor, Marie read all the books on sex in English, French and German in the British Museum, and then read her own way through English law. She filed her own nullity petition in the Probate, Divorce and Admiralty Division of the High Court of Justice in October 1914, although the case, which was successful, did not come to court for almost two years.

Since 1912 she had been conducting a love affair with the translator and her biographer Aylmer Maude, but her love had waned by the time she met Humphrey Roe, then engaged to Ethel Burgess. Marie and Humphrey were secretly married on 17 May 1918, three weeks after Humphrey had signed a declaration to Ethel, which was accompanied by a lump sum of money, that he would not marry for six months. The ceremony was conducted by an old admirer, the Bishop of Birmingham, and Aylmer Maude gave Marie away. Dr Binnie Dunlop, secretary of the Malthusian League, who had introduced them, was Humphrey's best man. Everything had gone Marie's way and the marriage seemed to hold out the prospect of happiness at last. No wonder she appeared radiant at the time of her initial meeting with Helena.

Marie was academically brilliant; in 1905 the youngest doctor of science in the British Isles, a botanist with specialist training in fossil palaeontology, and uniquely experienced in the field of fossil coal. She was a lecturer in botany at University College in London, but the burning interest in her life was sexual reform, and she waged her campaign with relentless vigour. To this end she had written *Married Love* (1918) because, as she noted in the preface:

In my own marriage I paid such a terrible price for sex-ignorance that I feel that knowledge gained at such a cost should be placed at the service of humanity.

She expected the book to electrify England, but she had considerable difficulty in finding a publisher. Stanley Unwin was willing to take it, but his partner did not wish to. Eventually A. C. Fifield accepted it. He was prosecuted and heavily fined on publication, but by the autumn found himself with a best-seller on his hands, and was complaining that he could not fill all the orders he received. It eventually sold over a million copies. The *Lancet* and *British Medical Journal* both published favourable reviews of *Married Love*, but omitting any reference to birth control. George Bernard Shaw told Marie it was the best book of its kind he had ever read, but *The Times* returned its review copy as 'hardly suitable'.

Helena had read *Married Love*, and was broadly in agreement with the message that Marie was delivering with all the force of her own frustration that the woman must be concerned in the physical side of marriage. Marie believed that

> Women must be taught how to regain the instinctive delight in physical passion that society had succeeded in repressing, and that men must learn to recognise these unacknowledged needs and to substitute for immediate sensual gratification a greater understanding and sensitivity.[1]

The book contained medical mis-statements, antagonised the Catholics and enlightened thousands, including the young Naomi Mitchison, who as Naomi Haldane had been married in 1916.

> It told you the basics, the sort of things everybody knows now, which had been firmly kept from us. When I got *Married Love* it was such an eye-opener I rushed out and got a second copy to send to Dick, who was liaison officer with the French in Italy, and said, 'Now read this before we meet again,' which he did. I didn't know much when I married at eighteen. It just made all the difference.
>
> Personal communication to the author—11.2.82

Marie followed up *Married Love* with *Wise Parenthood*, which was published later the same year not, as she was to infer, as a response to

[1] Ruth Hall, *Marie Stopes: a Biography*, Virago (1977).

84

demand following *Married Love*. She already had the manuscript of *Wise Parenthood* with her in Cornwall, which she asked Helena if she would read. Marie had by now become convinced that birth control and sexual technique were indivisible, and maintained this concept in the face of opposition by her friend George Bernard Shaw, who was to tell her in 1928 that she was 'really a matrimonial expert which is something much wider and more needed than a specialist in contraception'.[2]

Helena and Marie discussed the medical and contraceptive aspects of *Wise Parenthood*, and as Helena has said:

> I told her I would look at the manuscript provided she gave me *carte blanche* to take out all the nonsense. No one had ever before suggested to Marie she could write nonsense, but she accepted what I had to say, and listened, surprisingly, with proper scientific interest. She showed at that time a deferential attitude to a much younger medically qualified woman. When I handed back the considerably mutilated script I was prepared for storms. None came.
>
> Personal communication to the author—3.5.81

After their Cornish interlude the Wrights returned to 49 Great Cumberland Place, still looked after by Lady Alice Leslie. The idea of the Chinese mission field was uppermost in Helena's mind and she began a preparatory period of post-graduate training in gynaecology, having found a Norland nurse for Beric. She went back to the New Hospital for Women, attended Louisa Aldrich-Blake's out-patient sessions and her ward rounds, and watched her operate. Peter, meanwhile, settled down to work for higher surgical qualifications. He had a good brain and passed without difficulty the examinations for the Fellowship of the Royal College of Surgeons and the Mastership of Surgery of the University of London.

The following year, 1919, Helena learnt that a medical missionary, Dr Harold Balme, whom she had met in London at the time she signed her Student Volunteer card promising to work in the mission field, was in England on a recruiting drive. He was now Principal of the Shantung Christian University in northern China, which he had founded fifteen years earlier. The university had reciprocity with McGill University in Montreal as well as a strong American link.

[2] Ruth Hall, *op.cit.*

Helena arranged for Peter to meet Dr Balme, explaining in her forthright fashion that they both intended to come and work in his hospital as medical missionaries. His response was to pull out a notebook with the intention of identifying a missionary society which had vacancies to fit the pattern that Helena demanded, herself as a gynaecologist, her husband as a surgeon.

It appeared that the Society for the Propagation of the Gospel filled the bill, but it was denominational, and Peter had been raised in a family of Plymouth Brethren, which might interfere with Helena's plan. He obligingly offered to join the Church of England and to be baptised. So off they went to Tufton Street in Westminster to interview the general secretary of the SPG. Taking the lead as usual, Helena asked to be part of the Society's missionary quota with her husband at Dr Balme's unit at Tsinan-fu. The conversation, according to Helena, went thus:

> SPG SEC Do I gather, Mrs Wright, that you're going to help your husband?
> HELENA No, you don't. You gather I'm going to have a job of my own as assistant gynaecologist. No midwifery, please. I don't like it.
> SPG SEC Our mission wives don't at present have positions in the hospital.
> HELENA Then you'll just have to change your rules. Either we both go and work, or neither of us goes.
> SPG SEC *after a pause*, You will have to see our committee then, and convince them.
> HELENA Of course, delighted, but on condition that I see each member separately in their homes. They only make cowards of each other *en bloc*.

Armed with the list Helena found she already knew many of the committee members, including 'Billy' Temple's mother, whom she had met with other ladies at the SCM conferences she had attended as a member of the executive. The battle, if there was one, was already won. It only remained to agree the terms. The Wrights' joint salary was to be £300 a year, and the SPG would find accommodation for them to rent—at Helena's wish, a Chinese dwelling rather than a foreign missionary house. It so happened that part of a Chinese estate comprising three courts was available.

Henry Lowenfeld agreed to subsidise the SPG salary with another

£500 a year for five years and Alice Quicke offered to pay an extra annual sum of £100 for the fare and services of an English children's nurse, thus enabling Helena to work in the hospital. Typically, Helena rationalised her mother's contribution: 'I didn't see why you shouldn't help your grandchildren if you wanted to' (HRW to AQ—Peking, 26.2.22).

In discussions with Helena over her allowance her father explained his promise to pay her £500 for five years, but not for a longer period:

> . . . One never knows what might happen and I don't want to take a firm engagement for longer . . . You ought to be quite clear in your expectations as to the future. At your mother's death you are safe to come into over £1,000 per annum, and at my death there is every possibility that there will be something left for you. But life is so uncertain and money does burn so in one's pockets that there is no knowing as to this. If I do leave something you will get your fair share, but if I should turn prodigal or go into stupid speculation I might have dissipated it all before my death and come to you and others for support. In fact all is possible.
>
> HL to HRW—Paris, 6.4.21

In the event that is exactly what happened. Towards the end of his life, and against Helena's advice, her father invested the bulk of his assets in the land of his birth and was caught by the devaluation of money in Germany and Austria after the war. Henry Lowenfeld died in Paris on 4 November 1931 in comparative poverty, leaving £419.5.8d. gross in England, as certified by probate on 6 April 1934: 'the net value of the personal estate amounts to nil'. Two months before his death Henry wrote to 'My darling Ellie' acknowledging the 'support' she had evidently given him:

> . . . Please do not fail to explain to Peter that the question of the overdraft was *entirely* your proposition. I should never have proposed it. For the war loan offer my *sincerest* thanks . . .
>
> All my love, kindest regards to Peter. Kisses and embraces to every boy equally.
>
> Your own Papa
>
> HL to HRW—Royat-les-Bains, 13.9.31

The arrangements for their departure for China took longer than Helena expected. This gave her the opportunity for a climbing holiday with Tom Hill in the Swiss Alps. They set off from Mürren and slept in a mountain hut on the Jungfrau, where Helena experienced mountain sickness for the first time. They then went on to Venice. Helena left the train at Milan to get a sandwich in the station; the train went on without her and she had to follow Tom and her luggage on the next one. Her holiday with Tom set the pattern of independence of one another where holidays were concerned which Helena and Peter were to follow all through their marriage.

By the time all the arrangements had been made for the Wrights' departure for China their second son Christopher had been born, on 18 October 1920. He was six weeks overdue which annoyed his mother. He was delivered, like his brother, at 49 Great Cumberland Place by the same woman doctor. As before, Peter gave the anaesthetic to his wife and, as before, Helena reproached him with not having provided her with a daughter. All he said was, 'I gave you what was good for you.'

It was not until 11 October 1921 that the party, including the children's nurse, Joyce Harpham, set off by train to Marseilles, breaking their journey to spend a fortnight in Paris with Henry and Frania. They then joined their steamship, a Japanese cargo vessel, the *Kitanu Maru*, at Marseilles. The Harold Balmes, together with their four children, were travelling on the same boat. They had reached Ceylon by Christmas, which they spent in the Galle Face Hotel. Then on, via Singapore and Hong Kong, arriving in Shanghai on 16 January 1922.

[7]
China Base

Helena and Peter Wright went to China with the intention of staying there for life. In the event the assignment lasted five years. These years made a lasting impression and turned out to be, in Helena's own words, 'a complete fulfilment of all I expected and more'. She found China the most beautiful country she had known, and she loved and admired the Chinese—with reservations. Peter and she proposed to 'live our own lives with our own unconventional ideas' at the Shantung Christian University, as missionaries, but the word 'heathen' was not in Helena's vocabulary.

She was a Christian, but not religious, and had been baptised, confirmed and married in the Church of England. Her beliefs were strictly personal,. and on her ninetieth birthday this is how she described their 'long evolution and change' in a statement for the press:

> My loyalty to a membership of the Church of England is mostly latent. I regret on its behalf the general absence of teaching and experience in its views (if any) on the nature and purpose of personal life after death. I welcome and join societies or groups who are actively seeking the re-emergence of the powers of healing, spiritual, physical, and psychological, promised by Jesus and fulfilled by the Apostles. As these promises long antedated the formation of any organised Christian 'churches' I expect to find evidence of such healing in any of the present varieties of organisations labelled 'Christian'.

Helena may not have been able to express herself with such clarity sixty years earlier, but apart from a growing belief in an afterlife which developed with the years, it is doubtful if her views changed much from those she held as a missionary in China. And what an improbable missionary this unconventional young woman made!

Her definition of a missionary differed from that of her father, with whom she had some altercation of a semantic nature while discussing her future plans. He insisted that she was 'full of false ideas' and would 'come down to earth' when she had lived with 'real missionaries' for a year or two:

> Missionaries are maintained by charity, and *they* must also contribute by rendering their services at the very barest means of subsistence . . . and if people ascertained that their money was being used by *fully* paid missionaries they would certainly instantly stop contributing. The word 'missionary' implies sacrifice. The wildest stretch of imagination can not call you, as you propose to do it, a 'missionary'. You are just as much a 'missionary' as the child of rich parents is a 'workman' when he enters a shop to learn a trade.
>
> . . . There are some people who pass all their lives in the sky, but they are almost invariably people who have no wants, while your wants are many, and worst of all your ideas raise rather expensive hobbies . . .
>
> H L to H R W—60 avenue du Bois de Boulogne, 6.4.21

Henry went further and warned her that people like her did 'a *vast* amount of harm' in mixing with 'real' missionaries, and that as a result no one could tell who was or was not a 'real' missionary, all of which he foretold would lead to bitterness in the minds of the 'true' missionaries. None of his arguments, of course, deterred Helena who seldom changed her mind once she had decided on a course of action. Nor did it deter her father from making her the allowance he had agreed. Even with this she was sometimes short of money in China to meet the living standards she expected to keep up.

As for being a 'true' missionary, again Helena held her own views. She knew that missionaries were expected to spread the Gospel, and that their fellow missionaries would hold evangelical beliefs. All they were in China for was to preach. But she and her husband were not preachers or proselytisers; they were going to work according to their own lights, for the good of the Chinese.

> We were Christians, but not talkative Christians. We were prepared to answer questions and to enter into an argument, but not with the idea that we had the answer to life, although we had our own answer. If the Chinese wanted to know our answer all they had to do was to get to know us better.
>
> Personal communication to the author—31.12.79

Peter's views were more realistic, as he explained to his mother-in-law when they had been in China for over a year:

> I think educational work is missionary work; in fact it is one of the most important branches of it now-a-days. Most of the evangelistic work can be done by the Chinese so much better than any foreigner can possibly hope to do it; firstly as they rather resent being talked to by foreigners and prefer their own people, and secondly they understand the Chinese so much better than they do us. The object is to make the Chinese churches self-supporting and confine the activities of foreigners mainly to organising and teaching . . . Our job is to turn out Christian doctors, teachers, pastors etc who will do much more effective work than any number of foreigners.
>
> P W to A Q—Tsinan, 30.9.23

Hearsay evidence suggests that, as Henry Lowenfeld had forecast, not all her fellow missionaries, particularly their wives, shared Helena's views, and Helena admitted that this sometimes led to gossip and social difficulties, usually associated with her relationships with the Chinese or even other missionaries' husbands.

Before the Wrights could put their ideas into practice they had to learn to communicate with the Chinese. They spent their first year learning Mandarin at a language school which an earlier American missionary had founded in Peking. They and the Balmes were met at Shanghai and taken to a hostel for the first few days. They set off from the quay in a cavalcade of rickshaws, each child sitting on the lap of an adult. It amused Helena to hear the conversation between three-year-old Wykeham Balme and his father who, in spite of prodding the rickshaw coolie, failed to make him change course when directed. 'Daddy, he's not alive,' said the little boy, who had not been in China since he was a year old. Eventually they arrived at 'Missionary House' where Helena found to her surprise that all the Wrights and Joyce Harpham were expected to sleep in one big room, something she had never done in her life, even at school, but which appeared quite usual for missionaries.

Helena thought Shanghai the ugliest city she had ever seen. Her first impressions are preserved in a letter to her mother, the first of her weekly letters from China:

We arrived in Shanghai early on Wednesday morning. It was a brilliant, cloudless day and the place looked its best, which isn't saying much.

The surrounding country is absolutely flat, unbroken by anything whatever except a few, low trees so there is no charm of situation. Coming from the boat by rickshaw, what struck me most? The varied, but universal, ugliness of the buildings: they really are appalling. The European houses are all built of an inharmonious mixture of brick, red and blue-grey, the Chinese ones seem to be made of complicated rubbish. The next impression was the tremendous number of people that crowd every space: if a nation's strength lies in its population, China won't ever be beaten. The people *swarm*, and I can understand scoffers wondering why anyone bothers to preserve the sick. . . . To me, the chief ideas called up by a Chinese street, so far, are restlessness, and a complete absence of dignity or sense of form. It's all intensely interesting, but not beautiful at all. There is nothing that could be called architecture.

HRW to AQ—Missionary House, Shanghai, 14.3.22

The Wrights spent five days looking round the various hospitals and colleges in Shanghai, and Helena was agreeably surprised to find the missionary enterprise larger than she had anticipated. Her judgement of Harold Balme was vindicated when she discovered in what respect he was held after his fifteen years in China, years in which as a single-handed missionary he had first come across an isolated missionary station at Cheeloo. This he had amalgamated with two other stations, creating a university with three faculties, Medicine, Theology and Arts. He was now the Principal and Professor of Surgery in the Faculty of Medicine of the Shantung Christian University at Tsinanfu. In China he had met and married his wife who was a 'real' missionary, as Henry Lowenfeld would have described her, of the evangelical persuasion.

The line to Peking runs north from Shanghai via Nanking, where the Wrights were met on the next stage of their journey by Jim Wallace to whom Helena had once been briefly engaged. She found Jim older and looking rather sadder, perhaps, she wondered, regretting he had not followed his original intention of becoming a missionary. He was now working for the Sun Life Assurance of Canada in Nanking. Helena throughout her life managed to keep in touch with her numberless friends; her links with Jim had been maintained and were to be continued in China after his marriage. Jim saw the Wrights over the Yangtse River, over a mile wide at Nanking in its transition to the deltaic course. Here they changed trains and continued north-wards, stopping on the way at Tsinan-fu where they were eventually to work once they had completed the language course. At Tsinan-fu they stayed as the guests of two missionaries, Jocelyn and Eileen Smyley, while they fixed up their accommodation and work for the time when they would return from Peking. Their departure for Peking was delayed because the entire family, including Joyce, got influenza in the Smyleys' house, but at last, after a journey of over six weeks, they arrived at their destination.

Helena was enchanted by the wonders of Peking, which they explored by rickshaw or on foot. She was indignant at the sight of the ruins of the Summer Palace, north-east of Peking, looted by Euro-peans who in 1900 had come to save the missionaries at the time of the Boxer Rebellion. They saw the marble boat on the lake, which it amused Helena to know had been built by the Empress with money allocated for the reconstruction of the navy and was now a functionless tourist attraction. She took the little boys to the Imperial City where within its six miles of enclosing walls was the Forbidden City with its golden-yellow tiles in which, under Manchu rule, no Chinese might spend the night. They went to the Temple and Altar of Heaven in the Outer City, where the Emperors spent the night on the eve of the Chinese New Year. She showed them the Bell and the Drum Towers and where they could hire boats and picnic on the North and South Lakes. She was entranced by the brilliant colours of the flowers, azaleas, rhododendrons and peonies, by the flowering trees, the waterways and the museums with their priceless porcelain and tapes-tries.

There were over two thousand foreigners in Peking, but the Wrights relied for their social entertainment on their fellow mission-aries, among whom there were Americans, Scottish, Irish and Welsh, 'a splendid lot' she called them.

Their real kindness and friendliness to one another is a constant pleasure. Here you get naked family life, just fathers, mothers, children all equally sharing in the troubles and work of bringing up offspring; there's nothing to soften the rubs and jars, and yet I've never met so many truly united families, or husbands and

wives so genuinely devoted to each other. It's certainly true that
money, luxury or externals do *not* make happiness.

HRW to AQ—Peking, 1922

Helena found the missionaries quite different from the 'society' of
Peking which was to her as 'bad as Cheltenham'. When invited to a
formal dinner for twenty at the British Legation she was contemp-
tuous of the formality with which they were served English food by
Chinese waiters, and vowed she would never go again.

Helena was delighted with the Chinese house they rented in Peking.
It was reasonably furnished and built around two walled courts into
which a gateman locked them at night. Four single-storey buildings
were arranged on the points of the compass, so that the entrance on the
north led to their living-rooms on the south side; the guest room and
sleeping quarters looked east and west. Every room led directly into a
court with no other communication between the rooms. The Wrights,
far from grumbling at the inconvenience in cold weather, found this
arrangement an amusing part of Chinese life.

Helena acquired a cook, who marketed and supplied meals as well
as cooking them, and paid him 2/6 a day for each adult, 1/3 for Beric
and nothing for Christopher. They found an *amah* to help Joyce, and
took on two 'boys'. Only the cook spoke any English. With three
words of Chinese, and no shopping experience, the arrangement
suited Helena admirably, who, as she described herself many years
later, was 'the same miserable housewife that I am now'. She saw the
cook's face as 'a mountain range of wrinkles, with all the wiliness and
good nature of the East', and had the sense to leave all negotiations
with him to Peter, as the man of the house.

While she hated Shanghai Helena felt quite differently about
Peking:

> The little streets, *hutungs*, are characteristic and completely
> un-European. Each is lined with a blank wall on each side about
> 12 feet high. The walls are pierced at long intervals by the gate-
> ways of the compounds in which the Chinese all live. Only when
> the gate is opened is the interior visible. The doors are often
> very fine massive blocks of wood, painted bright red or dark
> blue with shining brass handles of Chinese shape, mostly round;
> the imposing rooflets are heavy stone tiles with decorated eaves.
>
> A motor practically fills up all the *hutung* which is about ten
> feet wide. When my bicycle and I see one coming we cling to the

side wall with the fewest bumps near it. The great feature is the street sellers. They are mediaeval and of endless variety. Each man carries his wares or apparatus at both ends of a long bamboo pole balanced on his shoulders. Every trade has its own sound. The barber twangs a fierce tuning fork, the sweetmeat man uses two little brass trays like castanets, the knife grinder has a long English-sounding hunting horn; others have loud chants, and so on.

They all perform all the time and the combined sound in the otherwise noiseless city is extraordinary. We sit here in our living room trying to decide what it is like, but Europe has no parallel. Blind men play on guitars, as they walk, haunting delicate little tunes. The streets have an endless fascination. Every here and there a *hutung* will break out into little shops all made of carved wood, one storey high with paper windows and fantastic hanging signs. Sweet water wheelbarrows are everywhere; they are very heavy and make the weirdest squeaks from their axles. That sound haunts my dreams; the Chinese love it, but there are no words to describe it.

HRW to AQ—Peking, 1923

It was along these streets that Helena and Peter would bicycle daily to the language school. The classes were small, with six to eight students in each. There were two sessions a day, morning and afternoon, from which they would return, in Peter's words, 'like a damp rag'. In practice the system was an efficient one, designed by a former missionary, whereby they learnt syllable by syllable in each of the four tones, each with a different meaning in Mandarin. Nothing could be written down; the teacher illustrated every word in pantomime, but never by direct translation. As Peter described it: 'The teacher holds a pencil or a book or something, and makes a noise somewhere in the middle of his chest which we endeavour to reproduce more or less inadequately.'

They learnt five new words in the first half-hour of every day. The group would then move to another teacher, who would make conversation using the new words grafted on to those already learnt. Every half-hour the teacher would change and another would continue the conversations. It was a good practical method which followed the principle whereby a child learns to talk without learning any grammar. Each pupil made his own picture of what he was learning, and just as no two pupils saw the same picture so they differed in skill, but not in standard. They learnt nothing about Chinese characters and Helena decided she would not attempt to learn written Chinese characters anyway, but Peter was captivated by the language and eventually became more proficient than Helena. Helena loved the many Chinese expressions: to 'flatter' was to 'give the person a tall hat'. The first day of spring was 'the day the insects wake up', and the first day of winter, 'the day the butter won't spread'.

Evidently they both made good progress:

> After five weeks we have learned over two hundred words and can use them all in conversation. Everything depends on the order of the words. To get at that order there is nothing to help; it's just a feeling to be acquired by instinct and ear. Knowing other languages is not a help except as practice in expressing your ideas. The teachers know no English, but are trained to explain everything in simple Chinese with action, and all have a subtle sense of humour.
>
> HRW to AQ—9.3.22

Helena and Peter would practise their new skills on their servants, who listened politely and were then apt to break into a vacant smile, which made the Wrights wonder how much progress they had actually made. When later on they had to teach Chinese students they at first used an interpreter, but by December the following year Peter was able to give his first lecture in Chinese at Cheeloo, an experience he told his mother-in-law he found 'rather a painful proceeding' and modestly thought the students must have been 'very intelligent indeed to get anything out of it'. The following autumn Helena gave her first lecture to students and was then able to conduct their oral examinations with only two corrections by her co-examiner. But Helena was never one to rest on her laurels. At the end of the language course someone said to her, 'So you've finished learning Chinese?' to which she replied with her usual feeling for words, 'I've finished being taught, but I've not finished learning Chinese.'

(above) *Student days at the Royal Free Hospital. Dr Harrington Sainsbury, flanked by his junior doctors. Back row, Ward Sister, Staff Nurse and students. Helena is on the far right. 1911/12.*
Photograph Royal Free Hospital archives.

(right) *War wedding, Chapel of the Savoy, 17 August 1917.*

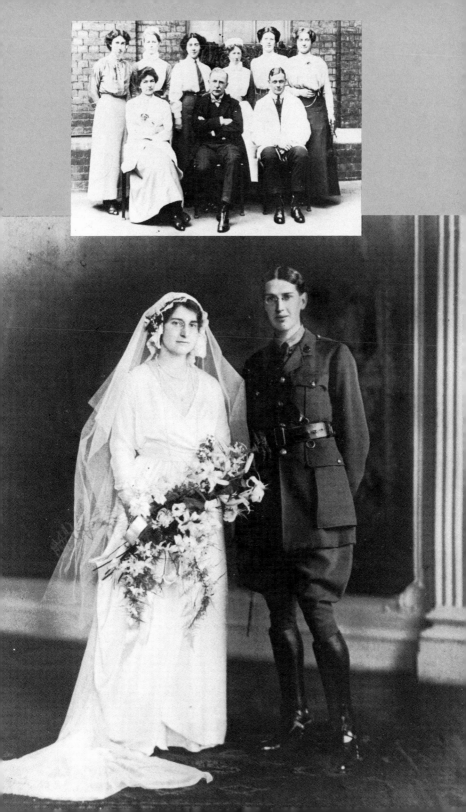

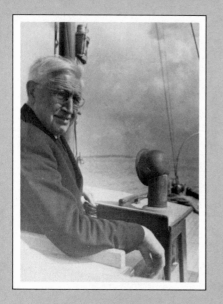

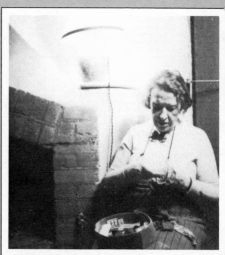

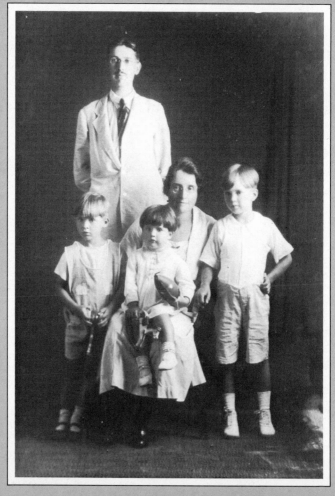

In the spring of their year in Peking the Wrights had a break in their language course and spent a week at a World Student Christian Federation Conference at Tsing Hua College six miles north-west of Peking, to which Helena and Peter had been invited as delegates. Helena was enormously pleased to have been invited, remembering the 1913 Conference of the wscf at Lake Mohawk. She told her father she felt doubly privileged, and how much the Christian testimony, particularly of the Indians, impressed her.

The Wrights had arrived in China when antagonism to all foreigners was on the increase, and particularly towards the British whom the Chinese believed supported the hated Japanese—while Germany had been locked in conflict in Europe in the First World War the Japanese had seized German property in China. The collapse of the Boxer Rebellion in 1900, in which thousands of Christian converts and over two hundred foreign missionaries had been slaughtered, led to heavy reprisals and was a bitter success for the foreigners. The far-reaching humiliating effects of the Boxer treaty affected all the big towns, imposing restrictions on Chinese control of the main services, Customs, the Post Office, railways and the administration of the important salt tax. When the Wrights were in Tsinan for instance, a Dutchman was responsible for the salt tax, an Italian for the Post Office. The Boxer treaty gave foreign legations land which belonged thereafter to the foreign country and not to the Chinese, and on which the foreigners could and did build houses forming a foreign enclave. Resentment against this extraterritoriality was a major issue during the time the Wrights were in China.

Another factor which impinged on their life was the continuing battles of the war-lords between 1916 and 1926. The 1911 revolution transferred power from the last emperor when the country became a republic, but it remained divided, as competing generals sought to

(left) *China c. 1924. The Doctors Wright with their three eldest boys.*

(above right) *Margaret Lowenfeld (1890–1973), children's psychiatrist with an international reputation. Henry Lowenfeld said: 'Madge has the brains and originality, Helena the capability.'*

(above left) *H.W.S. (Peter) Wright, dedicated surgeon and a magistrate; a pessimist with a streak of melancholy in his nature, interested in music and the arts. 1951. On board his pride and joy, the 'Cairngorm', a refuge from the complexities of life.*

control the country. The Wrights witnessed the effects of the break-down of the national government prior to Sun Yat-sen's return to power as president in 1923 until his death in 1925, and the launching of Chiang's northern expedition in 1926.

They found themselves in the centre of the civil war soon after their arrival in Peking. As foreigners they felt secure, while they watched from the sidelines the 'incredible mixture of comic opera and savage tragedy', enacted by the two main factions, those of General Wu Pei Fu and General Chang Dso Lin, and the army of the puppet government which opposed both sides. The soldiers were amateur mercenaries, according to Peter, 'The last person who wants to fight is the soldier if he can possibly desert and steal civilian clothes, poor devil.' If they lost a battle they were apt to change uniforms and put on spare badges belonging to the winning side, Peter told his father-in-law in April, when describing the local situation. But the following month the comic opera had developed into something more serious:

> Last Saturday the familiar sound of heavy gunfire began. Things developed slowly. Peking was put under martial law several days ago, and as the police and some troops have actually been paid up to the day they really will defend the city. Last time in 1920 there were separate rioting parties in the west, east and north quarters of Peking. Each time soldiers were sent to control the rioters they did so and then themselves entered another quarter and began looting on their own, to be quelled in their turn. This time they are doing it better.

> Every Chinese knows that the foreigners won't be touched, so they do their best to pretend *they* are foreigners. The rickshaw boys even put Union Jacks or American flags on the rickshaws. This afternoon heavy rifle fire suddenly broke out quite close to us. Our servants were scared grey, rushed to the compound gate where they tied a small Stars and Stripes to the post! This evening a friend brought the explanation. Wu Pei Fu is said to have routed Chang Dso Lin, and put his soldiers to the run. Wounded are streaming into Peking and the hospitals are getting full. Peter has been given a surgical team at the Rockefeller Hospital. We were summoned there last night and did two operations. Peter had the knife and I gave the anaesthetic. Next time it's going to be the other way round.

> Trains between here and Tientsin have stopped because both

sides have portions of the line. A train load of soldiers came up to the city gates and tried to get in. Peking defenders on the wall opened fire and killed the engine driver, many men, and took six hundred prisoners. Rumour says the dead and dying are still lying outside the gate.

In the meantime ordinary life goes on as usual. Inhabitants are warned not to be out after 10 p.m., and the enormous city gates are closed at about six o'clock.

HRW to AQ—Peking, 5.5.22

The closure of the gates seems to have been the only hardship suffered by foreigners, who could no longer attend evening meetings because half the community lived outside the wall. The Wrights had by now learnt to detach their minds from the decapitated heads mounted on poles on the wall, and had had to come to terms with Chinese brutality.

But by June the Wrights had become more closely involved in the civil war. General Wu Pei Fu, after a much bigger battle, called on the Peking Union Medical College, formed in 1920 by the Rockefeller Foundation, for help with over three thousand wounded at Paotingfu, a town four hours by train from Peking, where there was a small American missionary hospital. Helena and Peter were only too delighted to join the rescue team. 'Doing our real work is beans to us,' was Helena's reaction. The language school was after all only a means to an end.

A special train was sent from Peking for the team which included two Scandinavian nurses and three Americans, who were bringing an X-ray plant and equipment, transported in accompanying covered vans. A short way out of Peking the train stopped and a soldier brought a message that one of his mates had hurt his leg. The Wrights climbed out and there on a stretcher lay a man with one leg crushed to pulp from knee to ankle. The bones were exposed and the foot was hanging by a few muscles. Helena described the experience when writing, as she had promised, to Joyce Harpham, looking after Beric and Christopher in Peking while their parents were away:

Keeping the man alive with no apparatus of any kind occupied us all for the rest of the journey. It was very hard to get a decent tourniquet on to stop the bleeding. At last I succeeded in borrowing the chief Chinese official's walking stick. At 3.30 in the morning we arrived and waited on the platform until two ruffians and another stretcher turned up accompanied by a policeman. We mobilised all the boys standing about and made an absurd procession about twenty strong, sleepy, dusty and cold, the man on the stretcher only just alive, our lantern throwing weird shadows. We set out on foot down the railway line and off into China, stumbling in and out of deep ruts, anxiously seeing that none of the luggage disappeared.

At the hospital all was in darkness. The only porter asked who we were, and we eventually got the patient into the theatre to have his leg off. At 5.15 I sank most gratefully into bed and slept until 8. That day we worked hard. The hospital is packed with wounded, no rubbish and all dangerously wounded. They have given us a ward each with responsibility for all the operating —glorious. We did seven operations between us this afternoon and are now so dead tired I can scarcely think. The whole thing seems so ridiculously familiar, the wounds look just like European ones, the smells are the same, the difficulties the same . . .

The operating theatre has two tables going, patients being brought in as fast as the last one's bandages are put on. Dr Lewis, the head man, has been operating from morning till dark every day since the rush began and is pretty tired. So is the other man. They are very pleased to have us and we are delighted to get at our own job again.

HRW to Joyce Harpham—Paotingfu, 9.5.22

Peter's experience in the war in Europe stood him in good stead, as he told his father-in-law:

It was a very funny and in many ways a heart-rending experience to do war surgery again. I found the people there making all the mistakes we made with our cases at the beginning of the last war. The old boy in charge who was old enough to be my father would no more believe me than become a Mohammedan fakir. I suppose no one will ever learn from anyone else's experience till the world ends . . . I think in the end he saw from our results. In the week we were there he did four amputations, and while our cases were similar we did not have to do any at all. The soldiers were much like ours in essentials, very docile and most grateful, cheerful and irresponsible. They all made up their minds that once they got into hospital they were going to die, and those that didn't were correspondingly surprised.

It was a great triumph that the Chinese themselves asked for foreign help and did all in their power to make that help effective. They seldom call on foreigners in that way. In spite of the fact that their hospitals were in the same city they sent us all the bad cases. This took a great deal of persuasion as they thought we would bag all their cases to preach to, but as we treated them with the strictest professional etiquette they gradually got over their fear of losing face and came along.

One day Wu-Pei-Fu himself turned up and we showed him his hand under the X-ray. He was very bucked when he saw a bullet in a man's face and then the man from whom I had removed it. We told him the hospital wanted an X-ray plant of its own and he asked how much it would cost and we said 60,000 dollars [8 Chinese dollars then equalled about £1]. He said 'buy one and send me the bill'. This was very appreciative of him as it was quite disproportionate to any expense the hospital was put to over the cases.

PW to HL—Peking, 12.5.22

Peter then explained to his father-in-law that the lesson he had gained from this exercise was the importance of knowing the language. Few foreign doctors spoke Chinese well, but if only missionaries could talk to the rich Chinese, of whom there were many, he believed their educational efforts could be made self-supporting. 'Rich men will give generously when we can prevent them looking down on us.'

By the following month the civil war seemed to have petered out, though no one knew if an armistice had really been signed. Chang Dso Lin had given back some of the rolling-stock he had stolen, and one train a day was running to the coast at Peitaiho. Peitaiho was important for the missionaries in Peking because there they had a number of holiday or rest houses where they could escape the summer heat. By June Peking had become uncomfortably hot and the language classes began earlier in the morning. The students did not go back in the afternoon, but collapsed in the heat at home.

Shortly after the Wrights returned from their mission to Paotingfu Peter noticed that for once, and contrary to his usual experience, Helena was more tired than he was. She had a high temperature and developed a rash which turned out to be scarlet fever. This illness upset her considerably: she was not used to being ill:

It certainly is thoroughly beastly being ill, but here I am after
sixteen days in bed sufficiently recovered to be allowed to write
my first letter. I've been lucky to have a light attack, and
yesterday my temperature for the first time stayed normal all
day. Peeling goes on very rapidly; it's all finished except legs,
hands and feet. My hands look as if they were covered with some
cheap material which is wearing out. Scarlet fever is desperately
virulent here and people used to die in six hours before the rash
came out, so it is much feared. Luckily no one caught it from me.

HRW to AQ—Peking, May 1922

At the end of that hot and rather difficult summer the Wrights
decided they would stay on at the language school for another term.
After this they moved down to Tsinan. By then Helena had again
become pregnant and was referring to the baby as 'Rosamund'. She
paid no attention to her father's advice 'also to fix a boy's name, as to
my mind there is every reason to suppose that it will be wanting', as
indeed proved to be the case. Helena was pleased that 'Rosamund' was
to be born in March, which would be a 'good month for this climate,
neither hot nor cold'. They had found the last summer in Peking very
trying, particularly Peter, who felt that with the possibilities of more
war casualties, he could not get away to Peitaiho with Helena.

It was winter by the time they arrived in Tsinan where the
temperature was arctic and the ground frozen to a depth of eighteen
inches. Before leaving England Helena had sold much of the contents
of Great Cumberland Place, and the remaining furniture had been
crated and sent by sea to Tientsin. The Wrights had rented another
Chinese house in Tsinan, and moved in on 19 January 1923. In
addition to thirty-three packing-cases from Peking, Helena now had
the crates of furniture from home to deal with. For a fortnight she
laboured with painters and carpenters for the whole of every day,
talking to the workmen in what she described as her 'villanous'
Chinese. Three rooms had only mud and brick floors and Helena had
the bright idea of covering them with the wood of which the crates
were constructed. Hai, the carpenter, discovered to his amusement
that the wood the packing-cases had been made of, which was 3/4-inch
in thickness, had come originally from China, a land short of trees
where wood was therefore scarce. He imagined that Helena had
deliberately returned it to his country and he became her slave. He
happily laid her floors, and copied, with the proverbial Chinese skill,

her Chippendale furniture in such immaculate detail as to be indistinguishable from the original. He framed from the same wood the enormous canvas of a landscape she had brought from London. It was the size of the mattress of a double bed and looked well over the Chippendale sideboard in the dining-room.

By the time Helena had finished she had created what she considered the best of the foreigners' houses. It had four single-storey buildings which all opened into a large garden, and, as in Peking, no room communicated with another directly, so in winter anyone, including the children, wanting to move from the sleeping to the living quarters had to put on fur coat and ear muffs and go outside. There was of course no central heating, so Helena had three stoves built into the house. One of these heated the bath water, normally brought in from outside in buckets, and she devised an ingenious scheme by which a tank inside their bathroom wall conserved hot water by a form of insulation which would have done credit to her friend Tom Hill, now an architect of some distinction.

Their landlord, a rich elderly Chinese merchant, lived on the other side of the wall that enclosed the estate. He and Peter became good friends, and whereas Helena might be invited to 'welcome tea', their Chinese host insisted on giving Peter Ovaltine, when he came to visit. As in Peking the servants included the all-important cook, two boys, and an *amah*. The cook knew a little English, cooked ordinary English food quite well, and Chinese dishes if required. Again Helena left the accounts to Peter. The table boy served the meals, set the table, cleaned the dining-room, did the fires, brought the bath water, helped in the kitchen, and could, when required, put on a white coat and wait at table. The *amah* was Helena's prize, a sweet elderly Chinese woman who was a Christian, with tiny bound feet, who did the children's and Helena's washing and helped Joyce with the children, especially Christopher who was already proving a handful. According to Helena his will was already fiercer than his brother Beric's:

> If Christopher wants anything he screams the roof down and will not be diverted. Yesterday he stood at the door and yelled without ceasing the whole afternoon because he was not allowed into the court where a sandstorm was in full force at the time.
>
> HRW to AQ—Tsinan, 13.4.23

The gateman was married to the *amah*, and whereas the other servants lived in three rooms leading out of a courtyard 'reminiscent of a stable

block in Poland', as Helena described it, the *amah* and the gateman
had their own quarters by the gate in the eight-foot outer wall.

> The cook is very tidy and dignified, speaks slow and beautiful
> Pekingese. Apparently there's nothing he can't do, from putting
> up hooks to darning holes in my umbrella. He keeps the court
> tidy, brushes it with Beric's help and waters all the flowers. He
> answers the telephone, brings the letters and does all the jobs
> that turn up . . . They are all pleasant people and seem happy
> with us.
>
> HRW to AQ—Tsinan, 27.2.23

Tsinan was a walled medieval city, with four gates manned by
soldiers and closed nightly. It was a rapidly growing commercial
centre, with rail connections north to Tientsin and Peking, south to
Shanghai, and east to Tsingtao, a seaside resort which had been developed by the last German emperor. The hospital was within the city wall,
but the university with the medical school was a short distance outside. Harold Balme had designed the campus buildings for the three
faculties when he first arrived at Cheeloo. There was a library, lecture
and seminar rooms, and a chapel, as well as some housing accommodation for the staff. The administration block was important, and
contained the equipment for the translation and printing of textbooks
into Chinese.

The community in which Helena and Peter now found themselves
was divided into two camps, missionaries and business people. The
European business people lived in what was known as the 'Settlement', and employed servants who spoke English, and were in
consequence better paid than the missionaries' servants. Missionaries
spoke Chinese with their servants and paid them less. But one servant
who applied to Helena for a job in her household told her he preferred
to work for her rather than in the Settlement, because he knew he
would never be struck by a missionary.

Helena was not by nature socially inclined, and she already had
good friends in the Balmes and in other missionaries, Dr and Mrs
Robin Mosse, whom she had also met in England and who were now
back at Cheeloo. The Balmes and the Wrights remained friends after
their return from China. According to members of the Balme family,
Mrs Balme had reservations about Helena as a missionary, and
Wykeham Balme admitted to being, like many others, 'intimidated' by
Helena; but their eldest son, later Professor David Balme, CMG, DSO,

DFC, saw her for the last time when she was over ninety and found Helena 'still the same warm, alive, lovable woman and full of ideas as she had been in China'.[1]

Helena soon discovered that even if she was hardly a 'real' missionary she preferred the missionaries in Tsinan to the business people. However, even with the missionaries Helena came in for some criticism. None of their wives were professionally employed, except for running the Foreign School where Beric, and later Christopher, were pupils, and where Helena taught hygiene once a week. Helena was aware that, as the only woman who smoked, she attracted a fair amount of adverse comment, apart from her unorthodox views, and her attitude to the Chinese, who could enter her home uninvited, and through the front entrance, which one missionary wife told her was 'unwise'. But, of course, to no effect. Helena merely regarded this attitude as supercilious.

On their arrival from Peking, Peter had found a Chinese teacher, who came every afternoon to teach him the Chinese characters. He therefore worked in the hospital only in the mornings at first. Helena's pregnancy stopped her from working at all in the hospital at this stage, but word got round that here was someone who could fill a gap. When she was over seven months pregnant she was called on to operate on a girl with acute appendicitis, with whom she had shared a house at Peitaiho the previous year. A less stalwart character might have left the job to her husband, who had, of course, much wider surgical experience than Helena, the gynaecologist, but this evidently did not enter Helena's head. Peter was also in demand.

> People soon discovered how indefatigably industrious Peter is and work him accordingly. My life when it is normal will be much the same, except that I already get a large proportion of foreign women as patients. Ten of the wives of English and Americans have been to consult me already.
>
> HRW to AQ—Tsinan, 27.3.23

The Wright's third boy, Michael, was born on 10 April 1923. Helena had arranged for an American woman doctor 'to usher Rosamund into this sunny world'. When they arrived in Tsinan Peter had told his wife that this time she really would have to be looked after by a male doctor. 'I certainly shan't,' said Helena, and once more got her own

[1] Personal communication to the author—7.6.82

way, but she admitted that finding a woman had been difficult and, when success crowned her efforts, it had been a 'weight off my mind'. Qualification for the task ahead was a minor consideration compared with her sex, although the doctor herself raised the question of her suitability; but to Helena the over-riding importance of gender won the day.

Like his brother Christopher this baby was several weeks overdue. Helena wondered again if post-maturity ran in the family. Although her mother had told Helena she had weighed twelve pounds at birth, hardly possible except in the case of a diabetic mother, she could never find out from Alice the exact duration of this pregnancy. Helena was quick in complaining about what she called her 'third failure' in a letter to her mother:

> Isn't it disgusting about the baby? Three boys, nearly as bad as the Lowenfelds. But he really is a darling. I like him much more than I did the other two as infants . . .
>
> HRW to AQ—Tsinan, 15.4.23

She found Michael 'the most adorable baby in the world' and frequently referred thereafter to his 'lovely smile' and 'engaging dimples'. Her father, who had received a monosyllabic wire on 11 April, 'BOY', offered his crumb of comfort:

> . . . My wife rushed in today with the telegram in her hand. As there was one word only we were reassured . . . You can imagine my joy. Do believe me I feel very pleased.
> . . . You wanted a girl. One can never tell what is the best, but quite frankly for the child's sake I prefer a boy. They are harder to bring up, but if they come out right their lives are so much easier.
> I am dieting, viz keeping on low rations, but tonight I will drink your health.
> Love to Peter, to you, and the children and to the new Baby.
> Your own
>
> Papa
> HL to HRW—60 avenue du Bois de Boulogne, 11.4.23

At this point in her reproductive life Helena decided she hadn't the courage to risk a fourth pregnancy. She was happy with her three boys as she later wrote to her unmarried sister:

To have three beautiful sons, one as exquisite as Michael, is indeed a fine, soul-filling experience. Why not try it?

HRW to ML—Tsinan, 25.5.24

After Michael was born Helena decided that she should learn to look after a baby entirely by herself. She took him to Tsingtao, once a German settlement, two hundred miles away where the missionaries would rent or share summer cottages at Iltis Huk, a rocky promontory with beautiful bays, purple islands and golden sands two miles out of the town. They could sail, and picnic and swim from the long sandy beaches.

From this time all Helena's letters to her father which have been preserved show an increasingly loving relationship between father and daughter, in strong contrast to the acrimonious exchanges between Helena and her mother. Many letters which began 'My darling Mother' contained a barb of varying intensity—thus:

. . . One or two points apparently want further emphasis. In writing or thinking about you, I don't *judge* you at all. I have at last thoroughly realised that it's not one human being's job to judge another. I was trying to tell you the impression the facts of my life made upon me, willy nilly, with no judgement in the matter.

I have always, since as far back as I understood anything, thought of you with profound pity, can you guess on what grounds?

(1) Because the fairies at your christening forgot to give you a sense of judgement, and this has dogged you all your life. You never seem to be able to choose rightly, or to be able to gauge people's characters. For this reason you have been the sport and plaything of your circumstances.

(2) There is something really weak in your character which comes out in such remarks as that you wouldn't have married Frank if Madge or I, or anyone, had said a word against him. I can't imagine such a state of mind. If the world, and my family, had talked against Peter, I should still have relied on my own judgement of his worth, and married him without a qualm.

Given these two various disadvantages, life hurled you into *very* difficult circumstances, which anyone with sound judgement and a strong character might have found extremely hard to manage. I am certain that you always thought you were doing the best possible thing, and spent your last ounce of energy in trying to do it. So please, Mother darling, feel and understand that you have my fullest sympathy with your unhappy life. I only wish I could help you. Frank worries you every day, he hasn't the slightest right to be supported by you without doing any work, and yet you won't send him away, and save his character by making him work—that is the sort of way *your* character makes you a continual slave. With your certain income, and circumstances free from *real* worries, you ought to be happy and contented, but you aren't—which brings me to the third reason why I have always pitied you—the fact that you were born with a worrying and unhappy nature, and were never taught that a tendency to worrying absolutely *must* be controlled if any peace and happiness is to be attained . . .

Now—do you understand a bit more? What I want you to see is that our present relation is a direct result of our past, considering the difficulties of our two characters, and your policy during my youth. I don't think a child has much choice in its feelings towards its parents, it is largely in the hands of the parents. If my children aren't true friends with me when they grow up, unless they turn out thorough bad characters, I shall know that it is my fault, and not theirs.

. . . As to the future, it is still largely in your hands. I am perfectly willing to be friends, if you can realise that we are two grown-ups, and if you will give up wanting to 'influence' me and give me advice—I would always rather make my own mistakes, and learn by them, advice is no use to me. Of course the very biggest thing you could do, would be to take yourself firmly in hand, and kill the grievance habit. You and your sisters have the same attitude to life, you all go about looking for slights, hurts and grievances.

HRW to AQ—Peking, 7.6.22

There is no evidence that poor Alice ever took Helena's advice but perhaps she was mollified by a letter she received later from her son-in-law, who had by then been married to Helena for nearly five years. Peter's letter reveals interesting aspects of his as well as Helena's character.

Dear Grannie

. . . I want to try to say something about your relations with Helena which perhaps will make you happier. If I say anything which is critical please do not feel that I mean it in this way. I feel very strongly that unless you face certain ordinary facts inherent in any maternal relationship, you will never find a basis for friendship. Unless you do so, I am sure Helena, at least, when she gets a great deal older, will regret it very sincerely.

Now the fundamental thing which upsets you about Helena is that you have not the least influence in determining her course of action one way or the other. You also feel that you ought to have, and that in not deferring to your wishes, or consulting your opinion in any of the major issues of her life she is doing your love and care for her a great injustice.

Now Helena is a rather exceptional person, in some ways, but not nearly as exceptional as she thinks she is, and as her environment has led her to think. What she has got is exceptional executive ability, but it has not very often been worked off on her equals, usually on her intellectual inferiors, round whom she is accustomed to make circles when she wants her way. If she had constantly to deal with her equals in ability many of the corners would have been wiped off and she would soon realise that the BULL BY THE HORNS policy is not the one which cuts ice in those quarters.

. . . At 32 or so she has had in her life much more responsibility and much more experience than most women . . . and on the whole has carried it off very well, considering her lack of training for it . . . Here is therefore rather an exceptional situation which we have to control . . . Everybody in this modern world will rightly or wrongly take their destiny into their own hand after a certain age. The only thing you and I can do is to stand by Helena with a glue pot and pick up the pieces when trouble comes. We shall then find that respect for the glue holders increases with time instead of diminishing if the glue is put on with a loving hand.

. . . I feel I have said enough about this and I hope you will not feel I have done wrong and am guilty of impertinence.

We all send our very best love.

Peter

PW to AQ—Peking, 29.5.22

By early summer Peter was working hard at Cheeloo. He was responsible for seventy surgical ward patients, held out-patient sessions and taught students. He was still finding the language a problem. He was extremely interested in his work, and in the students who were drawn mainly from the agricultural community in which the university was situated. He regarded the students as highly intelligent on the whole, although he was rather surprised when one of their number came to ask him if he could modify his report on a student who, his colleagues feared, was not appearing to do well. He, Peter, was learning to understand the Chinese:

> The governing classes are corrupt to the core. The middle and student classes intensely patriotic and the lower classes have all their work cut out to get their food and elementary necessities of life . . The student classes take themselves very seriously and work very hard and are most willing to make friends with anyone who will meet them on terms of friendship and not drop seeds of a superior culture from the heights of an Eton and Oxford manner. Their friendship is wonderfully worth having, as they seem quite straight when they trust you. Their motives are just as simple as ours are when we take the trouble to sift them out. We find a curious absence of the inscrutability which all the books talk about. Their hospitality is boundless.
>
> PW to HL—Tsinan, 28.4.23

The Wrights found themselves in a culture which over the ages had venerated learning, in which scholars were rated above politicians and where the military, who fought not for pay but only for food, came lowest of all in the hierarchy. They watched with admiration as their students changed under their eyes from peasants off the land into critical and conscientious doctors, in accordance with their cultural veneration for education and scholarship. The students' ascent in the social scale, which their degrees and qualifications had established, promoted an egalitarian relationship between themselves and their teachers.

Few foreigners made friends with Chinese students, but the Wrights' pupils came regularly to their home, where the doors were always open to them. On one occasion Helena found a boy sitting absorbed in contemplation of the large Leader landscape. 'Is this what England is really like?' he asked. 'All those trees?' Helena was gratified when three fourth-year women students—women were in the minority—invited her one day to lunch in the 'Women's Dormitory'. They ate solidly from 2–4 p.m.

A young Chinese doctor, Hou Pao Chang, became a regular visitor to the Wrights' house, and with him Helena and Peter formed a lifelong friendship. They had known him in Peking, where he had graduated at the Peking Union Medical College (PUMC). His father was an aristocrat, one of the last graduates of the indigenous Chinese university, 'The Forest of Pencils'. His son's education began at the age of four, when the child was required to learn four Chinese characters a day, and continued thereafter on purely classical lines, relying entirely on rigorous memorisation, so that by the age of ten the boy was a Chinese scholar. At this impressionable age he heard a 'foreign devil' talking in Chinese to a group of villagers. The speaker was an inspired, proselytising missionary, a Dr Cochrane who noticed the child on the outskirts of the crowd and encouraged him to join his school. Hou Pao Chang saw a new world opening before him, and went on to become a doctor and eventually professor of pathology at Hong Kong University.

He held a junior appointment at Cheeloo after leaving the PUMC, and the relationship between him and Peter became one of devoted pupil and teacher. His affection included the family of the teacher and particularly the young Michael. Before long he announced that he wished them all to use a special name for him—'Fu Lin'—which signified 'Always Returning'. Sometimes he would return to help Helena with difficult Chinese words when she was due to give a lecture to the students. Once he returned to help her with a domestic problem, when a quantity of sheets mysteriously disappeared. They were good, valuable sheets and the Wrights could not afford to lose them. What to do? Fu Lin said, 'Nothing. Wait.'

A week later a deputation of five unknown, well-dressed Chinese gentlemen arrived to see Peter by appointment. They were carrying antique porcelain jars. Having introduced themselves they announced that they had heard rumours in the city that certain sheets were missing from the house; these rumours touched their honour, as they did Peter's. They had a proposition to make, which turned out to be that the Wrights should forget about the sheets and accept their gift of porcelain jars. In his best Chinese, Peter explained that impecunious missionaries much admired Chinese porcelain jars, but had not the cash to send to Europe for linen sheets. It was too much, he felt, to accept such valuable gifts from the honourable visitors. They bowed and filed out and the sheets miraculously reappeared, all faces saved.

Soon Helena was working as hard as Peter, teaching students, and operating on gynaecological conditions once or twice a week as required, and sometimes doing general surgery, harelip and breast operations. She removed an enormous fibroid on one occasion, and the museum curator mounted the specimen. On an Open Day of the university a visitor passing through the museum noticed the giant tumour, and immediately and correctly recognised it. 'Ah,' he said, 'that can only be from the inside of Mrs X, who now has no swelling of that proportion.'

Although she was later to make her name as an authority on family planning there was no call in China for this field of gynaecology at the time Helena was working at Cheeloo. Infant mortality was so high that nature controlled family size. Helena would ask her patients how many children they had had, only to find that most women could not remember. They might offer the number as 'six or seven'. But when Helena had learnt to ask how many *living* children a woman had the answer would usually be one or two.

Peter quickly learnt that the Chinese philosophy with regard to illness was unlike that he had encountered as a student and young surgeon in England:

> It is lucky that most of their diseases can be diagnosed by merely looking at them. Talking becomes an accessory and is only necessary in persuading them to be treated. Their minds easily grasp the fact that a disease they can see should be removed. But where nothing is visible the great talk begins. But before any course of treatment, an X-ray or an operation, is to be embarked upon I am up against the system which has kept China an entity for the last thousand years—the family. They must all be consulted. Often they live 300 miles away. The father whom the patient is supposed to support calls in the village doctor and all the family come to the conclusion we are getting the better of them. They very naturally refuse and the patient never appears again.
>
> One passes to the next bed, a man with cancer of the tongue, say, with glands of the neck involved. The growth gives him much pain, especially when indulging in his favourite pastime, drinking tea . . . Yes, he is prepared to have the growth removed. He will think about the lumps in his neck when he is

better from the tongue and they are bigger. You embark on a long explanation of why they are the most important of all and must be done first. He will consult his father tomorrow. All this must take place without the least impatience or any show of trying to persuade. If you give him a hint that you badly want him to take a course of action he is right off the idea. It is then absolutely certain in his mind that you are getting something out of it some way or another, and out he goes.

The diseases are so advanced by the time you get them that the operations are very formidable indeed, and one hesitates before undertaking some of them. Everywhere the money question is at the back of their minds and even the most enlightened ones will jump at the opportunity of doing you out of a bit. In all our dealings they think we are making money out of them. Consequently they also think they should get something out of us at every possible opportunity.

PW to HL—Tsinan, 27.2.23

Interestingly, Peter had noticed another difference between the attitude of Chinese patients and those he had encountered in Europe. The Chinese did not necessarily want a result which a European surgeon would consider a good or even an ultimately desirable one. The Chinese patient wanted a quick and an economic result. There were some conditions which every Chinese believed a foreign doctor could cure, among them bladder stones. In such instances the foreign surgeon would encounter no difficulty in carrying out any investigations he considered necessary. However, one man failed to behave in the expected manner. He had walked, as many did, for three days to the hospital with his wheelbarrow, but when Peter diagnosed a stone in the bladder the patient refused treatment. It transpired that his mother-in-law did not trust foreigners and had forbidden him to allow one to operate on him. Mother-in-law must be obeyed, and so the patient returned on the long journey home. Eighteen months later he came back to the hospital. By now the stones were considerably larger, but his mother-in-law was dead and he could cheerfully accept the foreign devil and all his works.

As time went on the people in the Settlement as well as the missionaries began to appreciate the Wrights as social assets at dinner parties. To please Peter Helena agreed to some social engagements, including bridge parties. She had never liked the game though, and had only played on the ship coming out to China because Peter liked to play. She much preferred chess, a game she continued to enjoy when she was well over ninety. She would not play Mahjong in China because she considered it gambling of which she strongly disapproved, and she would certainly not play bridge for money.

As part of the social scene Helena decided in Tsinan to try her hand at amateur dramatics for which she had proved to have a natural talent as a schoolgirl when cast as Touchstone. A missionary's wife in Tsinan induced both Helena and Peter as well as Joyce Harpham to act in *The Mollusc*, in which Helena played the lead as a spineless individual who was a tyrant in disguise. Helena emerged as a natural actress and the play was so successful that it was transferred to Tsingtao in the summer season. The Literary Society was entranced by her success and in 1926 gave her the lead in Shaw's *Saint Joan*, then playing in London with Sybil Thorndyke. Helena also joined the Choral Society and sang soprano in *The Crucifixion* with the choir at the Chinese church.

What she really enjoyed was the countryside and the mountains beyond the city wall. She would walk the six or seven miles over the plain on numberless excursions with other missionaries or their wives. Some would go by rickshaw, or by carrying chair. The Wrights built a bungalow at Iltis Huk with the proceeds of the sale of the Great Cumberland Place lease, and Helena would spend the hottest months of the year at the coast with the children. She had chosen a site on a rocky promontory which looked both north and south, and had the cottage built to her own design, remembering all the lessons she had learnt from Tom Hill. The holiday home consisted of a single-storey building with five verandas and playing space for the children. The sandy beach to the north was three miles long, and Helena would walk there in the early morning before anyone else was up. Donald Godfrey, a missionary to whom Helena was greatly attached, might be staying, and would join her on these early-morning excursions during which they would discuss every subject under the sun so that she learnt to understand the mind of another missionary.

Much as she loved the coast, the mountains gave Helena even greater pleasure, which she recorded in a letter to her mother after an excursion from Tsingtao with Robin Mosse and Harold Balme to the mountain Lao Shan—'The Old Mountain'.

We are just at the southern tip of the plain of north China, and the mountains are all to the south. We went out at first by carrying chairs, seemingly ramshackle devices with string seats and a foot rest. There are shoulder straps (for the coolies) of leather and rope at both ends of two carrying poles. You pad the chair with a rug and cushions and it isn't at all uncomfortable. Two men carry it and go at a fast walking pace.

We went by chair to the tip of the valley and then climbed down a path as steep as the entrance to the Yosemite. We then climbed slowly over two passes, then on to the bare brown top of quite a high hill and down the other side when we suddenly saw a narrow valley between the next two hills. Its sides were covered with little trees in flaming autumn colours, crimson, yellow and brown, every here and there varied with the sober green of Chinese cypresses. Going down was heavenly because we saw the colours at all levels and the sides of the valley were winding, making great blocks of clear shadow. At one end was a beautiful little temple, behind it a spring and to one side quite a big pool. We sat outside and had our lunch, and then went down the valley by the stream and curled down into the head of another valley just as beautiful. There the temple was built into the rock itself half way up the wall and had glorious views of valley and trees.

HRW to AQ—Tsinan, 19.10.23

The following month Helena made a longer excursion to climb the mountain T'aisha with her friend Mrs Lennox Simpson, an American pianist whose husband, a writer, worked on the *Far Eastern Times* for which Helena herself wrote an article about the 6,000-foot mountain considered sacred for three thousand years. She noted that the Pilgrim's Way, the P'an Lou, leads from the lower reaches of the mountain and consists of six miles of paved roadway interspersed with seven thousand very steep steps cut by centuries of pilgrims into the side of the mountain. The sides are lined by cypresses and every now and again there is a small temple with inscriptions on the walls. It took Helena and her friend five hours to reach the Jade Temple at the summit and three hours to come down.

That autumn Peter's mother came out from England to visit them. Helena was delighted and found her mother-in-law the perfect guest, because she made no demands and seemed happy all the time, settling into the new environment as if she'd lived in China all her life. She had barely arrived when the Wrights took the old lady up T'aishan. Peter heard the chairmen singing to themselves as they carried her between them: 'We have a very special lady with us, a foreign lady of many years. She has gleaming white hair which she covers with a hat.' Soon Helena, writing to her mother, felt her mother-in-law had been there as long as they had themselves:

> We get lots of fun out of her [Mrs Wright] . . . and of course she's endlessly useful in the house. We have started making the servants do out the rooms properly and she stays and watches them. Mrs Wright's method is to go on talking English with a fixed smile until they somehow divine what she means. Of course they treat her with the greatest honour; anyone with white hair in China is certain of respect from everyone . . . You would be bored to death here, but she seems perfectly content.
>
> HRW to AQ—Tsinan, 7.10.25

Her arrival was fortunate for Helena who had not been well for much of that year. In May she developed mumps, and two months later she had a sudden attack of amoebic dysentery. She considered the treatment, which she described to her mother, 'much worse than the disease':

> Every other day swallow Yatren powder every 3 hours for 6 doses. The days between have large cleansing enemas and Yatren 200 cc injected into the large bowel which has to stay there for the rest of the day if possible. Yatren is violently purgative so you can picture what a peaceful life I'm having. In the meantime I consume a miserable diet of slops and cereals, and it's so hot that most of the time my nightdress is dripping with sweat. The treatment is very lowering, so although I feel quite well I get tired very easily and my head swims, so don't expect much of a letter.
>
> HRW to AQ—Tsinan, 13.7.25

In December her liver was considerably enlarged, probably as a result of her amoebic infection, but she did not, as was feared, develop an amoebic abscess in the liver, which gradually subsided with weeks of further treatment. During this illness the doctor who was looking after her discovered that Helena was pregnant. Her reaction was typical:

You will be pleased to hear that we are making our fourth and last attempt at producing a daughter. She ought to be born in early October and if she isn't a daugher we will be speechless with rage. Four is more than we can afford but I want a daughter very much. If it is twin boys we will sell them, an easy matter in China!

H R W to A Q—Tsinan, 7.3.27

Adrian, the last of the 'Rosamunds', was born on 16 September 1926, the day before Helena's thirty-ninth birthday. The family had been down at Tsingtao until 10 September where, as she wrote to her mother, Helena had packed up the house, linen and blankets and unpacked them at Tsinan 'with extraordinarily little fatigue'. She went on to describe the events preceding her 'fourth failure' which did not, of course, leave her 'speechless'. That would have been quite out of character:

> Tuesday night I began taking drugs. Pains began more or less about noon on Wednesday and I felt beastly. At 2.30 we started injecting pituitrin with marvellous effect. Every now and then tho' the pains stopped dead, and when that happened we injected again. On Wednesday I had eight hours of them till midnight, then a dead time arrived and we scattered on to various beds and slept all was possible. At 9.40 the next morning they gave me the 4th and last injection; pains came on like the devil and stayed on until the unasked for infant was born at 11.30 . . . Madge will be interested in the action of my uterus, which was queer. The baby weighs 8lbs 5oz, has dark hair and blue grey eyes . . . Being one of our infants he is ideally good so far. Janet [Joyce Harpham's successor] can't understand why he never cries or fusses; he didn't stir all last night. Milk is appearing satisfactorily and I am so absurdly well that it's only willpower that keeps me in bed . . . Nothing makes up for his not being a girl, but I still have the grace to realise I'm an extraordinarily happy and lucky woman . . .

H R W to A Q—Tsinan, 18.9.26

Mrs Wright occupied herself in her usual helpful way with the new baby, and Helena returned to her work in the hospital sooner than she had done when her other children were born. The baby gained weight slowly. In October Helena told her mother that he had 'the temper of a fiend' but took the blame herself:

It's my fault, of course. I wouldn't try to work and feed him if it weren't absolutely necessary. It's not a good scheme.

HRW to AQ—Tsinan, 12.10.26

But a month later she reported that he was doing well and 'improving in temper'. By the time the child was six months old it had become apparent that he had sustained a birth injury, which left him with severe physical handicap as a spastic. His mother once told me that she felt her age at the time of Adrian's birth could have been responsible for his disability, about which she felt guilty. It is, of course, true that these conditions are more common in the children of older women, but with hindsight it is likely that the injections caused spasm of the uterus, thus interrupting the oxygen supply during the confinement —which would have been conducted differently today. Helena soon recovered from the disappointment of yet another son and after Adrian's birth life returned to comparative normality although there were already growing signs of impending exacerbation of the civil war, but this did not disturb Helena unduly.

I walked out yesterday beyond the campus and filled my soul full of the hills. Every day we have brilliant sunshine and every night stars shine like diamonds. It is a wonderful climate. When you think of us on Christmas Eve please be thankful with us that we are so very happy and contented . . . This country has got hold of us. I wouldn't leave it for anything permanently; its charm is endless.

A very happy Christmas to you Mother darling . . .

HRW to AQ—Tsinan, 1.11.26

For Helena Christmas was an eternal family festival, and every year in China she celebrated it as in London, in the Polish fashion which had meant so much to her father. Every year she managed to get hold of a tree which reached from the floor to the ceiling. It was always decorated and lit with candles. On Christmas Eve she provided the traditional large fish, even if it was not a carp. She searched the market for poppy seed for the pudding. She who had never cooked in her life taught the Chinese cook to make almond paste from Mrs Wright's recipe book. Past recriminations, the battles between warring parents and resentful children were all forgotten as the spirit of Christmas was rekindled every year by Helena. In Tsinan the Balmes often joined in the Wright celebrations and the memory of the splendour of the

Wrights' Christmas festivities remained with David Balme for sixty years.[2]

Christmas 1926 was to be the last the Wrights would spend in China. They were due to go on furlough the following January at the end of their five-year stint with the SPG. Mrs Wright would travel home with them. Helena and Peter had every intention of returning to China after their year at home, but since 1925 there had been warning signs that the position of foreigners might become untenable with the rise of the Nationalist movement. Sun Yat-sen died in March 1925, having reorganised the Kuomintang and built up an expeditionary force to subdue the northern war-lords. At Dr Sun's death from cancer in Peking Chiang Kai-shek emerged as the leader of the Kuomintang force. But two hostile rival 'Nationalist' governments were to operate in central China, Chiang from Nanking and the 'Reds' from Hankow. As the nationalist spirit increased there were student demonstrations in the streets of Tsinan and cries of, 'Kill, kill the Japanese', 'Kill, kill the foreigner', 'Kill, kill the British'. On 8 June 1925 during one procession when the students were on strike, Helena, who had gone out entirely unafraid to see what was going on, recognised a group of their Cheeloo students. They smiled agreeably at one another and one particular boy carrying a 'Kill the English' banner winked at her.

But the signs were plain and the Wrights had to consider what action they would take in the face of an extension of the civil war. Helena set out her proposals in a communal letter to her family which illustrates her dedication to the work in China which she had undertaken:

> I want to tell you now, while there is no apparent danger, and my ideas are unclouded by fear, how I feel about the whole question of leaving the country should danger to life suddenly loom up. Firstly . . . I do fully realise what mob action may be, and we don't minimise possibilities at all. Our first consideration will be, of course, the children, there's no sense or good in exposing them to danger, or even to definite risk. We are planning in case of necessity, therefore, to send them to Japan in charge of Janet Greening, to people of our mission or others, who would look after them indefinitely. We are going to keep a sum of immediately available cash probably in Tsingtao, enough to pay

[2] Personal communication to the author—7.6.82.

for their passages, so they can be shipped off at very short notice.

HRW to AQ, HL, ML—Iltis Huk, Tsingtao, 26.7.25

To her father Helena had written:

> I wonder how often people's lives turn out exactly or better than they hoped? Coming to China has been a complete fulfilment of all I expected or more . . . I don't seem built for life in the sunless machine-ridden West; it's so glorious in the East, and given a minimum of income so comfortable and happy. Do come and see it at least . . .

HRW to HL—18.1.25

The war did not, in fact, impinge on their lives before their furlough except as a nagging worry.

The family left Tsinan with Mrs Wright and the four boys in January 1927; the Balmes followed shortly after. Helena maintained that she intended to return to China in due course, and they left all their furniture which had later to be re-crated and sent on to England by sea. The crates in which the furniture had been sent from England came in useful. According to Helena it was only a matter of ripping up the floors in their rented house and remaking the original crates. Meanwhile they were bound for Moscow and eight days across Russia on the Trans-Siberian railway. Helena was a natural traveller. Before leaving she acquired a large Gladstone bag which she filled with oddments of material cadged from the Cheeloo community. She goes down in history, therefore, as the inventor of 'disposable' nappies. Adrian was kept happy in a hammock slung in their carriage, from where he could see the snowscape through the window.

They had got out of Tsinan only just in time. In 1926 Chiang had launched his northern expedition with 50,000 men; he had captured Hankow and set up a provisional government but was forestalled by the entrance into Nanking of other Nationalist troops who began to loot and destroy foreign property. By 1927 Chiang had driven out the Communists and himself proceeded to within two hundred miles of the province of Shantung. There he was obstructed by Japanese troops, but the Wrights had escaped the local Chinese battles with the Nationalist forces of Chiang Kai-shek, who reached Peking by June 1928, and formed the Nationalist Government in Nanking in October.

The Wrights' little party broke the journey home first in Berlin, and then in Paris where Henry had moved to a smaller flat in the avenue Henry Martin, his finances having deteriorated progressively since 1923. The old butler Kelly was still with him, Frania was welcoming and the reunion a happy one. Henry was concerned with the future of Chrzanow and suggested he should leave it to Helena. Wisely she saw the obstacles, and told her father she could not contemplate its administration. As a result it eventually passed in equal shares to her sister Margaret and Henry's niece Rösel Haberfeld (the daughter of Adolf who had looked after the estate), and subsequently to Rösel's son Till, who was the last owner, until it was annexed by the Communists.

It was not until Helena reached England that news of events at Tsinan reached her from Jack McCrae, a lecturer in the Theology School, who had moved to the temporary university headquarters at Tsingtao to try to keep the foreign members of the staff from a complete stampede out of China. Both students and staff had been terrified when they learned what was happening at Nanking.

In May Jack McCrae reported that he had had a visit from a member of the provisional Shantung Christian University Senate which was having difficulties with the Chinese staff and wanted him and the Treasurer to go back for ten days and help sort them out. Their Chinese colleagues were unwilling to carry on indefinitely, and were not prepared to announce the reopening of the schools in the autumn without some tangible proof of the foreigners' intention to return. Jack McCrae had already revisited Cheeloo once in spite of consular instructions to the contrary. He found things absolutely quiet, apart from the arrest of a senior arts student charged with Kuomintang sympathies, and the imprisonment of an ex-student. But the military news was confused, and three armies were evidently concentrating on the Wuhan cities.

McCrae could not further defy the consul and at Tsingtao he felt he had a good chance of persuading a considerable university force to remain to 'pick up the debris after the storm has passed'. In this he was justified, and in July he told Helena that a depleted staff had returned to Cheeloo. Harold Balme had by now resigned, but fourteen other members of the foreign staff were expected in the autumn, and he hoped that Helena and Peter would decide to rejoin them. Helena was an incurable optimist, but she had not by then decided either way. At the end of their furlough the SPG told the Wrights that the university had been taken over by the Nationalists and this tipped the balance. They did not feel justified in risking their children's future in the uncertain situation prevailing in China.

[8]

Home Again

The family reached England in March 1927 and went to stay with Helena's mother at Hounslow. Alice had assumed that they would spend their furlough with her, and mother and daughter had corresponded on the subject for at least two years before the Wrights left China. But, as Helena had warned her mother, the furlough was not an unqualified success. She and Alice had totally different personalities, Helena had always disliked the house with all its unhappy memories and found Frank Quicke as annoying as ever. She later described the year as a 'trying' one, but where else could they go? The elder boys went temporarily to a local day school. Helena found their reactions to England amusing with a few 'shocks', as when Christopher disobeyed her by turning a tap on a milk churn and maintained that the escaping fluid could not be milk because that came out of cows. Helena and Peter renewed old friendships; Peter spent some time at a surgical refresher course and Helena brushed up her gynaecology.

Helena clearly intended to return to China, although she had suspected that the Christmas before leaving might be their last there. But when the Wrights learnt from the SPG that there were no longer any jobs for foreigners in the hospital, it evidently came as a complete surprise. It is difficult to see why Helena had not envisaged this possibility, though it was not out of character for her to suppose that any course on which she embarked would remain open to her.

Peter was devastated at having to resign from Cheeloo. Pessimist that he was, he now said that going to China had been the mistake of his life. He had four children to support and although extremely well qualified and with teaching experience in China, his prospects in England were poor. He had voluntarily stepped off the young professional surgeon's ladder. Had he stayed in England he would have progressed via junior hospital jobs to specialist status. He had never really got on the ladder because he had gone straight into the RAMC on qualification and had not held any of the usual training appointments. After leaving the RAMC he had held a research job at the Royal Cancer (now the Royal Marsden) Hospital. The work he did there in the laboratory on the origin of a particular form of kidney tumour became recognised as the classical account of this tumour (hypernephroma), showing that this rare form of cancer arises in one definite area of the kidney. He had followed this up with a junior surgical appointment at the West London Hospital, but then went straight to China.

Now he found he was too academically qualified—MS, FRCS—to be acceptable in junior posts but, because he had not done the training jobs, he would not get senior appointments either at his own hospital, University College, or at the West London, or at any other hospital. No one on the selection committees knew how well he could operate and there was no one to give him any sort of testimonial as to clinical competence—except in China.

On their return he made an abortive and unsuccessful excursion into a general practice in the East End of London and then eventually became consultant surgeon to the German Hospital, to the Children's Hospital, Hackney Road (now the Queen Elizabeth Hospital for Children), Queen Mary's Hospital, Stratford, the French Hospital and other smaller hospitals. It took a long time to get these posts and compared with his peers this left him relatively junior in the professional hierarchy. Before the introduction of the National Health Service in 1946 consultant hospital work carried no salary and Peter depended financially on his private practice, in which he was not particularly interested, but he eventually made a reasonable living comparable with that of his wife.

Helena on the contrary had no interest in hospital medicine and no intention of improving her academic qualifications. She proposed to work as a private gynaecologist in London. In China she had heard nothing of the emerging birth control movement, but her mind went back to Marie Stopes and their meeting ten years ago. She realised that here could lie the solution to a problem of world importance.

Contraception was not in its infancy. The Dutch cap, originally known as the Mensinga Pessary, had reached England in the mid 1880s around the time of Helena's birth. It had been devised in the mid Seventies by a German anatomist, Dr Wilhelm Mensinga of Flensburgh, later Professor of Anatomy in Breslau, who was interested in the status and emancipation of women. The device consisted of a rubber disc with the rim reinforced by a watch-spring, which when inserted in the vagina occluded the opening of the cervix and prevented the passage of semen.

In Holland Dr Aletta Jacobs learnt of this through reading an article by Mensinga in a German magazine, and began a long correspondence with him in Flensburgh. Aletta Jacobs was one of the eleven children of a doctor in the north of Holland. Born in 1854, she had studied medicine in Gronigen and Amsterdam, and in 1879 became the first woman doctor in Holland, where women had not previously been admitted to universities. In 1881 she opened a free welfare clinic twice a week for poor women and children, and the following year she decided to add advice on birth control to prevent further ill health among her patients, using caps, condoms and spermicides. Dr Mensinga sent her samples and detailed advice on how to use his pessary, which she followed for about twenty women a week in her clinic, keeping detailed records of their case histories and clinical follow-up examinations in order to refute any possible charges on the harmful use of pessaries. Holland thus became the first country to practise scientific birth control on a large scale.

In England the first printed reference to the Dutch cap was made in *The Wife's Handbook*, which was to sell half a million copies when it was published in 1886. It was written by a Leeds dermatologist, Henry Arthur Allbutt, who intended it as a book 'which could be understood by most women, and at a price [6d] which would ensure it a place in even the poorest household'. It was a simple domestic manual on hygiene, ante-natal, pregnancy and baby care and contained one short chapter on 'how to prevent conception when advised by the doctor'. Spermicides were by then in mass production and Rendell's suppositories of quinine and cocoa butter were available in chemists' shops.

Sadly, the medical profession took offence at *The Wife's Handbook*, considering it 'detrimental to public morals'. Its very cheapness put it 'within the reach of the youth of both sexes'. The Royal College of Physicians of Edinburgh deprived Dr Allbutt of his licence and membership of the College, 'for having published and exposed for sale an indecent publication', and in 1887 the General Medical Council ordered Dr Allbutt's name to be erased from the British Register for 'infamous conduct in a professional respect' in publishing *The Wife's Handbook*.

Aletta Jacobs's birth control clinic had been the first in the world. It was followed by Margaret Sanger's clinic in America. In 1915 Margaret Sanger had visited Holland, where Dr Johannes Rutgers taught her the techniques for correctly fitting Mensinga pessaries, Aletta Jacobs having refused on the grounds that Margaret Sanger was not a doctor of medicine. She was a nurse, one of the eleven children of Irish immigrants. As a midwife in New York she had become aware of the poverty among large families with unwanted children and the consequent distress this caused. Defying America's Comstock Law of 1873 which made it illegal to disseminate information about contraception, on 16 October 1916 she opened with her sister Ethel a birth control clinic in Brownsville, New York. On the ninth day a disguised policewoman came, posing as a patient, allegedly for instruction, and returned to arrest Margaret. She was released on bail, immediately reopened her clinic and was re-arrested with her sister. She and Ethel were sentenced to thirty days in the workhouse. There Ethel went on hunger strike and was the first woman in the USA to be forcibly fed. Margaret's appeal against the Brownsville conviction was heard on 8 January 1918 and resulted in official re-interpretation of the law. Henceforth doctors in the USA could give contraception advice 'to prevent or cure any alteration in the state of the body'. For the next twenty years it was still technically illegal to send contraceptive material through the post, until Margaret Sanger's successful test case in 1926, which was only one aspect of her ceaseless activity in promoting the birth control movement in the USA.

But in spite of the work of these pioneers, even as late as the 1920s in England mothers might have as many as twenty children. Only about one woman in twenty of child-bearing age was protected at intercourse, usually with a condom, and most poor women relied on abstinence or *coitus interruptus*. Lack of information and embarrassment were formidable obstacles, and birth control was considered too disreputable even to mention in public circles. Around fifteen per cent of recorded maternal deaths followed abortion, or attempted abortion, and of every hundred children born in England and Wales, approximately five died in the first year of life.

Helena returned from China to find the birth control movement growing despite fierce Catholic opposition. Marie Stopes had become a national figure, though detested by the medical profession as well as by Roman Catholics, and by 1920 she had become a member of the National Birth Rate Commission. In March 1921 with her husband's help she had opened the first birth control clinic in Britain, in Marlborough Road, Holloway. Though her books were bitterly criticised by the medical profession, who found it outrageous that a botanist had written on medical matters, Marie had enlisted the support of a number of prominent figures, among them Arnold Bennett, H. G. Wells, Arnold Carpenter, Maude Royden and Dame Clara Butt. Acting on Lloyd George's advice to try to make birth control respectable, she had formed the Society for Constructive Birth Control and Racial Progress (SCBC) with H. G. Wells as a vice-president, after a public meeting at the Queen's Hall at which she put forward the concept that birth control was the key to racial progress and the creation of happy, healthy, wanted children. In the following year, 1922, she had also founded a medical research committee on which Sir William Arbuthnot Lane and other medical authorities served.

Marie called her clinic the Mothers' Clinic for Constructive Birth Control. Only five hundred women attended in its first year, and police were required to guard it from bricks thrown by Catholic 'enemies'. The clinic's secretary for nineteen years, Elizabeth Harrison, recalled later that many of the women whom Marie released from the fear of pregnancy would not give their names at the clinic or allow her to send them the news sheet which Marie edited and largely wrote herself, *Birth Control News*, for fear of being identified as members of the SCBC.

In China Helena had not heard of the turning-point in Marie's life, the writ for libel which she took out in March 1922 against the Roman Catholic, Dr Halliday Sutherland. In *Birth Control: a Statement of Christian Doctrine against the Neo-Malthusians* (1922), Dr Sutherland, a convert, had argued that contraception was being promoted politically as a class conspiracy to reduce the number of workers and therefore voters among the working classes. The case dragged on for two years during which the defence put forward the imputation that in her books Marie was advocating sex among the unmarried. Marie retained Patrick Hastings, but even her own solicitors advised against the action, which was heard before the biased Lord Chief Justice Hewart who found in favour of Halliday Sutherland. Mrs Harrison, in a television interview on BBC2 in 1969, remembered the interest the case aroused, with crowds outside the Law Courts every day. The jurors took Marie's books home with them at the end of the case, but left Dr Sutherland's in the court room.

Marie appealed against the verdict and in July 1923 Lord Hewart's judgement was reversed in the Court of Appeal by a majority of two to one. Marie got a paltry but significant £100 damages, half the cost of the action and the cost of the appeal. Backed up by the Church, Sutherland appealed to the House of Lords in 1924. There by four to one (only Lord Wrenbury supporting Marie) their Lordships, three of whom were over eighty, decided in favour of Dr Sutherland, ordering, mortifyingly, the repayment of the critical £100 damages with costs against Marie. Bernard Shaw, writing to Marie, described the decision as 'scandalous'. Though she reckoned the costs of the case at £12,000 the trial greatly increased the sale of Marie's books, however, and thanks to the publicity her clinic flourished. She was in demand as a public lecturer throughout the country and not only began training nurses in contraceptive techniques but herself set them examinations.

The war had not been waged solely by the Catholic Church. In February 1924 the Anglican newspaper the *Church Times* had come out with a leader calling for support for Dr Sutherland. Many years later this paper was to complain about Helena's views when in a medical students' journal she suggested that engaged couples might profitably experiment sexually before entering into the lifelong commitment to marriage.

When in November 1921 the Malthusian League opened the second birth control clinic in the country at Walworth, behind the Elephant and Castle, they took the precaution of calling it the Walworth Mothers' Welfare Centre—no reference to birth control. There were two clinics a week. At one a nurse weighed the babies and gave mothers some practical advice, whispering at the end, 'Would you like to know how not to have another?' and explained that there

---

(lower right) *Christopher Wright, February 1949, on the summit of the Weissflugh above Davos. Attractive, charismatic, with personal gifts he did not use, he thought summers were for sailing, winters for skiing, but at the end found no purpose in life.*

(lower near right) *Helena and her only granddaughter, Miranda, at Quainton in 1963.*

(above right) *Architect Oliver (Tom) Hill. Arrogant, selfish and egocentric, his long-standing friendship with Helena dated from their childhood and survived arguments and differences: 'I was the person who mattered most in his life.'*

(above far right) *Bruce McFarlane (1903–66), distinguished Oxford mediaeval historian. The Wright household was his elective home from 1939 until his sudden death. Helena shared with him Brudenell House, which she regarded as her home, and where she intended to die.*

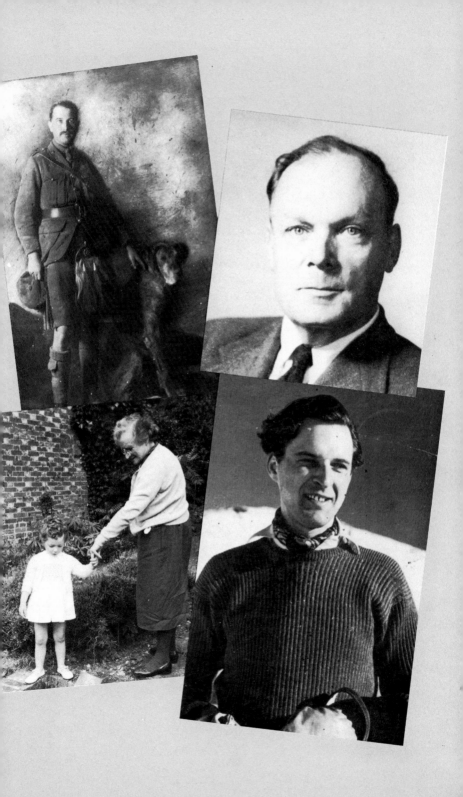

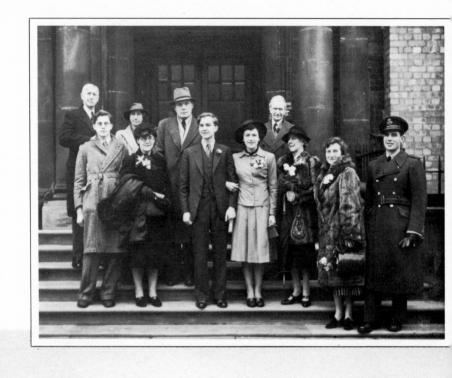

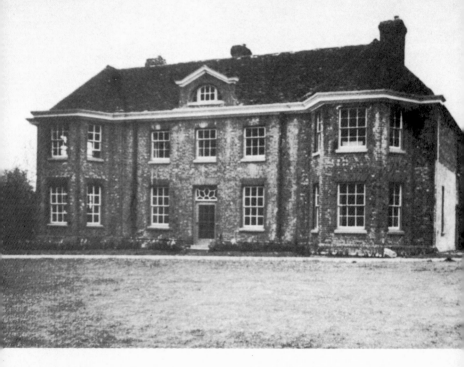

was a birth control clinic on another afternoon. Even so, there was the expected opposition, and eggs, stones and apples were thrown at the voluntary workers. Onlookers shouted, 'Whores', and 'Abortionists', laughed at the women who came to the clinics, and battered down the clinic doors.

The clinic ran out of funds because the women who attended it were too poor to pay for their appliances. The link with the Malthusians was severed and Walworth became purely a birth control clinic, run by a committee of voluntary supporters. One of these, Mrs Cecily Mure, has described the continuing Catholic opposition and how a priest told one Catholic woman who had thirteen children and had been warned by a doctor that another pregnancy could endanger her life, that she must burn her contraceptive diaphragm.

The campaign developed a new twist when political women became active and attempted to enlist Ministry of Health support. The Walworth Clinic sent a delegate to the Minister and Marie Stopes continued to press for birth control advice to be given at all maternity and child welfare clinics. She wanted to be the movement's guiding light but none of the political parties gave her any public support, and when a Labour government was elected in 1924, the new Minister of Health turned out to be Catholic. The senior Medical Officer for Maternity and Child Welfare at the Ministry, Dr Janet Campbell, reported that three thousand women died in childbirth each year but her report (*Maternal Mortality*, 1924) made no reference to birth control facilities. As late as 1926 the Minister refused to make birth control advice available in public health clinics on the grounds that doctors were not experienced in the work—hardly surprising since the medical curriculum included no instruction in the subject.

Meanwhile interest in birth control spread to the north of England. Mrs Charis Frankenburgh, a qualified midwife who had been at Somerville with another pioneer, Margaret Pyke, became increasingly concerned with the welfare of mothers and children in Salford and anxious about the practice of old wives' methods of inducing abortion, such as repeatedly jumping off the eighth stair when a period was

---

(left) *Brudenell House, formerly Quainton Rectory.*

(above left) *1940. The wedding of Beric Wright and Joyce Normand. Back row from left: Peter Wright, secretary Olive Stewart, Bruce McFarlane, bride's father. Front row from left: Michael Wright, Freda Bromhead, groom and bride, bride's mother, Helena, friend Roger Napier.*

overdue, or taking Beecham's pills. One woman from Salford she knew had had eighteen pregnancies, of which four children failed to survive, three were imbeciles and three miscarried.[1] In 1928 Mrs Frankenburgh wrote to Marie Stopes to ask who might be interested in helping her to set up a birth control clinic in Salford. Marie suggested Mrs John Stocks (later Baroness Stocks) whom Mrs Frankenburgh had known as Mary Brinton when they were both at St Paul's Girls' School in London, who was now also living in Salford. Accordingly the two got together with neighbourhood friends, formed a committee with Mary Stocks as chairman, Mrs Frankenburgh as organising secretary, and Mrs Robert Burrows as treasurer. Four months later, on 1 March 1926, they held the first clinic of the Manchester, Salford and District Mothers' Clinic for Birth Control with a capital of £190, and the support of Sybil Thorndyke and Lewis Casson. It immediately ran into Catholic opposition.

The hostile element was led by the Roman Catholic Bishop of Salford, Thomas Henshaw. As reproduced in the *Manchester Guardian* (22 March 1926), the Bishop's comments in the *Catholic Federation* urged the people of Salford to wipe out the clinic, which was unfortunately close to the cathedral, over a baker's shop where women might not be recognised as clinic attenders. The Bishop condemned contraception and the dissemination of sex knowledge among young people thus:

> Horrible things which formerly were scarcely ever spoken of by mature men and women are commonplace now for boys and girls. Eugenics—that wonderful science which aims at the improvement of the race by securing its extinction—has taught many to be tolerant of strange filthy things. The powers of evil have refined their methods and unsavoury subjects are clothed with scientific names. The promoters aim at something more than inculcating wrong principles and now they proceed to the opening of 'centres' where practical instructions may be given. One . . . has been opened recently not far from our Cathedral and I am told that people are flocking to it in great numbers. The police are powerless to put these teachers out of harm's way . . . The strange thing is that the fathers and mothers do not rise up in arms against those who dare to defile the minds of the people

[1] Charis Frankenburgh in a personal communication to the author—3.5.82.

and hound them out of the district. One would expect a hue and cry . . . I hope the time is not far off when the people of Greengate [will] chase it from their streets.

The local Catholic press bitterly attacked the pioneers as being 'well fed childless women foisting their abominable views on the unsuspecting gullible working class'.[2] The *Catholic Herald* (13 February 1926) then referred to Mrs Frankenburgh's shameless proposal to establish a birth control clinic and called her 'an impertinent busybody', condemning her 'unblushing attempt to introduce into Salford a form of legalised prostitution of marriage'.

The following month the *Catholic Herald* returned to the attack (6 March 1926):

> It would not be out of place to ask if Mesdames Stocks and Frankenburgh belong to the idle parasitic classes. Certainly their views are seconded with enthusiasm by those wealthy overdressed, childless, badly-bred women who throng the matinees every day and publicly flaunt cigarettes between their painted lips.
>
> The Catholics of Salford will hardly be doing their duty unless they make a vigorous protest against the abomination that has come into their midst—an abomination that, in Catholic eyes, is infinitely worse than the unnatural vices that were practised in the cities of Sodom and Gomorrah.

Tiresome as was the Catholic opposition at the time, Mary Stocks subsequently criticised the medical profession far more bitterly. 'After all, the doctors knew the conditions and few were prepared to help the women they had advised not to have any more children. They were the people I think were really reprehensible,' she said in a television interview on BBC2 in 1969.

This was the situation Helena found when she realised the future that lay in the field of contraception. Once she had made up her mind she went first to Marie Stopes whose Mothers' Clinic for Constructive Birth Control had moved to Whitfield Street in 1925. By then the numbers of women attending the clinic had greatly increased and Marie had published her *First 5000 Cases*. She greeted Helena warmly as a disciple and warned her against the spring-rim Dutch Cap or

[2] Mrs Stocks and Mrs Frankenburgh had seven children between them.

Mensinga pessary which Walworth favoured, and which Marie insisted would induce cancer.

Helena for her part was somewhat alarmed to find Marie so altered after ten years. Marie bitterly resented her lack of medical qualifications and insisted that her staff, as nurses, could establish better rapport with clinic mothers who regarded doctors with suspicion and associated them with illness. She argued that any nurse who could conduct a confinement could equally, with training, fit contraceptive devices and give the appropriate advice. This was not the only point of difference between Marie and her medical opponents. Marie knew no more medicine than in 1918 but, more significantly, as Helena now recognised, she was suffering from paranoia, though she certainly had reason to feel aggrieved at the actions not only of Catholics but of many doctors. Helena could see and hear the concentrated fear and fury engendered by the words, 'Roman Catholics'. She had allegedly once thrown the telephone across the room, shouting, 'Those Catholics again.'

Marie's first child had been stillborn—'murdered', as she said, by the doctors—but in 1924 the much-wanted offspring was born by Caesarean section. Curiously, just as Helena always referred to the child she was carrying as 'Rosamund', Marie equally wanted a girl and called *her* fetus 'Margaret'. She was soon convinced, when Harry Vernon Stopes-Roe arrived instead, that he was the most beautiful child ever conceived, and she was fiercely possessive about him, relegating his father to second place. By 1928, despite superficial appearances, her marriage was deteriorating and, ironically, barely survived the first edition of *Enduring Passion* (1928) which she had written at the age of forty-eight to give reassurance to the middle-aged, promising them 'lifelong love and enduring monogamic devotion . . . matured in a serene old age'.

When Helena visited Walworth she found women general practitioners were running the birth control clinics while the lay committee member, Mrs Cecily Mure, was looking after the administration. Helena had by then become convinced that birth control should become a specialty in its own right. At the North Kensington Women's Welfare Centre in Telford Road where Helena went next, she found an ally in Mrs Margery Spring Rice who with her Fabian friend Margaret Lloyd, a cousin of Bertrand Russell, had founded the centre, one of the earliest and largest of the voluntary clinics, on 6 November 1924. It was off Ladbroke Grove, once a fashionable residential area in London. Mrs Spring Rice had chosen it because by the Twenties it had deteriorated into a poor slum district with blocks of flats often without separate sanitary arrangements. When she opened the clinic there was still evidence of former glories in the Victorian stone blocks city gentlemen used when mounting their horses.

Margery Spring Rice, a 'promoter of lost causes' as she described herself, was widely involved in social and political reform as a Liberal and had organised the opening of the centre only six weeks after a committee meeting of some of her socially conscious friends who included the young Naomi Haldane, by now Naomi Mitchison. Margery Spring Rice came from a long line of feminist supporters. She was the daughter of Samuel Garrett, the son of Newson Garrett who, far ahead of his time, believed women had a right to a career, and she was also the niece of those indomitable sisters, Dame Millicent Fawcett and Dr Elizabeth Garrett Anderson. Her first husband Edward Jones had been killed in 1915 on the Somme and in 1919 she had married Dominic Spring Rice, the nephew of Cecil Spring Rice, poet and British Ambassador in Washington during the First World War. The marriage broke up in 1928, the year in which she and Helena first met.

Margery Spring Rice became secretary of the Women's Health Enquiry Committee formed in 1933 to 'investigate the general conditions of health among women, especially among married working-class women in view of indications that ill-health was both more widespread and more serious than was generally known.' It was the findings of the WHEC that revealed depths of social misery and injustice not previously imagined, and Mrs Spring Rice's contacts with patients at the North Kensington Women's Welfare Centre which stimulated her as secretary of the Women's Health Enquiry Committee to write *Working Class Wives: Their Health and Conditions.*[3]

At her first meeting with Margery Spring Rice Helena was able to convince her of the logic of her views that contraceptive advice should be given by gynaecologists specially trained for the purpose, of whom there were none in existence at that time. When next a vacancy occurred on the staff at Telford Road, Margery Spring Rice offered Helena the job, which she accepted on the understanding that she had a free hand to make whatever changes she wished. To Helena's

[3] Penguin Books, 1939; Virago Reprint Library No. 8, 1981.

surprise Margery Spring Rice agreed, and Helena worked as Chief Medical Officer at Telford Road for thirty years, becoming Chairman of the Medical Committee.

Through her the clinic became a training centre which attracted students, both nurses and medical graduates, from home and overseas. She made her international reputation on the lessons her patients taught her. Eventually the Centre became part of the Family Planning Association, but by then it was concerned with a wider field in addition to contraception. Sessions were held for both men and women in sub-fertility, marital and sexual problems, as well as pre-marital sessions and health examinations.

According to Naomi Mitchison, Helena had originally wanted the clinic to be mainly concerned with contraception, or birth control as it was then called, but the lay committee, including herself, was anxious to extend and broaden the services and eventually the committee won. Naomi remembered Helena in those early days as:

> . . . a short, round dynamic figure with bright eyes behind pince-nez glasses. She usually wore clothes with no concessions to any possible enhancement of her general appearance. She held very definite views and I enjoyed our meetings enormously, but I felt it was rather like swimming in a rough sea. Bounce! Bounce! We thought she was great fun, and all enjoyed our slight quarrels with her.
>
> Personal communication to the author—11.2.82

The arguments usually arose because Helena wanted things done her way and perhaps that was a reasonable approach on the part of the senior doctor, but it was also a facet of her personality, and even her devoted father had taken her to task on her inflexibility during a much earlier argument.

> Your logic and conclusions are all at fault, and if you had considered the matter from the other person's point of view and not only, as frequently, from your own, you would have saved me the trouble to write this letter which is far from a pleasant duty . . .
>
> HL to HRW—Chrzanow, 24.8.12

Naomi Mitchison found that Helena would not usually succeed in any controversy with Margery Spring Rice 'who was enormously competent, while none of us was entirely confident in those days'. For her part Helena appreciated Mrs Spring Rice and described her as an 'able and competent chairman', but Cecil Robertson, Mrs Spring Rice's only daughter, has spoken of the relationship between these two strong personalities as a 'mixed love-hate relationship', adding in a personal communication, 'They must have both been the least diplomatic women in history!' Her mother admired Helena's work but had difficulty in accepting her dogmatic and steam-roller approach, especially in sexual matters. She found it easier to work with another well-known gynaecologist, Dr Joan Malleson, who was in charge of the clinic for sexual difficulties at Telford Road, whose death from a drowning accident many years later, in 1956 on her way home from a visit to New Zealand, greatly distressed her colleagues.

Through her work at Telford Road Helena met various other sympathisers with the birth control movement, including Lady Denman and Eva Hubback, a Labour campaigner since the Twenties, Principal of Morley College for Adult Education and Chairman of the Workers' Birth Control Group (WBCG). Helena soon found herself in demand by other supporters of the mounting birth control campaign which by now included her old chief, Sir William Arbuthnot Lane as well as Arnold Bennett, H. G. Wells, Bertrand Russell and Julian Huxley.

She had become an acknowledged public speaker, her talent having been discovered by chance when, on her return from China, the SPG had asked her to speak to the Mothers' Union of Wiltshire and Dorset who had paid the Wrights' salary in China. The result was rewardingly successful and the mothers listened entranced as Helena told them simple everyday things about their domestic life in China: how the points of the compass were all-important; the serving boy would say he had placed various items of the meal on the east or west side of the table; about using chopsticks and how in the fields she had seen children adroitly trimming twigs to use as substitutes on the pattern of the simple genius of three thousand years. She described the flowers and the beauty of China. With her typically practical approach, she brought to the meetings little silk shoes to demonstrate the size of the tiny bound feet of her *amah*, four inches long, much smaller even than the size four which Helena, herself a small woman, wore. She spoke of the quilted coats and the layers of clothing which Chinese women needed in the cold weather—even in the summer the Chinese abhorred nakedness in any form and their clothes reached up to the neck and down to the ankle.

On 4 April 1930 a major public conference took place in the Central Hall, Westminster, at which Helena was asked to speak.[4] It was the outcome of the mounting pressure group campaign to get the Minister of Health to withdraw the ban imposed on public health welfare clinics from giving advice on birth control, the Ministry's argument being that such a sensitive subject could deter women from attending the clinics.

Delegates came from local and public health authorities, maternity and child welfare centres and from the pressure groups which included the Society for the Provision of Birth Control Clinics (SPBCC), the National Union of Societies for Equal Citizenship (NUSEC), the Workers' Birth Control Group (WBCG) and the Women's National Liberal Federation. Helena's friend, Mrs Eva Hubback, as Chairman of the Conference, proposed a motion to 'call upon the Minister of Health and Public Health Authorities to recognise the desirability of making available medical information on methods of birth control to married people who need it'.

As medical officer to one of the major birth control clinics in London which voluntarily provided advice which they could not get at public clinics to poor women who already had more children than they could afford, Helena decided to talk about the effect of education and training in contraception among the mothers she had taught for a year at the North Kensington clinic:

> The sort of women who came to our clinics were the real poor from the surrounding districts, all terrified as to whether or not the next menstruation would arrive, and all frightened of hospitals. They would come to us because we were all women, women doctors, women nurses, women running the clinic. They came to us without fear and in confidence that we could help them, which is of course what we did. I had the rewarding experience of watching a total change in their health and outlook.

Helena went on to compare this group of women with those uninitiated women who had provided Mrs Spring Rice with the material for her book, the women who lived with the haunting fear of pregnancy.

> Maternal morbidity is extremely widespread and enduring, so that a woman tends to become progressively less fit with the

[4] *Report of the Conference on the Giving of Information on Birth Control by Public Health Authorities* (London, 4.4.30), 17, 33–6.

birth of each child. Secondly, though some of the contributory causes of maternal ill health date back to childhood or adolescence, most of them are found in the conditions of the mother's present environment and work . . . The married working class woman is in a category by herself as regards the problems which concern the well-being of her family; not only because of the loneliness, isolation and primitive condition of her work, but also because her heart as well as her brains and hands is engaged in her labour.[5]

The examples cited by Mrs Spring Rice were typical of women who had attended Helena's clinics:

(1) Mrs E. R. of Bethnal Green, 43 years old, has had thirteen children of whom eleven, ranging in age from 24 to 1½ years, are living at home. She lives in a flat of three rooms and a kitchen, in a narrow, poor street. Her husband is a dustman and she has altogether £3.11s.0d. housekeeping money. There is no hot water and she has to go two floors down into the yard for her cold water.

(2) Mrs B. W. of Croydon, 38, has nine children, all of whom are living at home; the eldest is 10, the youngest are twins of 6 months. She lives in a small cottage of four rooms and a scullery but no bath. Her only complaints as regards her health are constipation 'on and off for twelve years', but this only occurs when she is pregnant or breast feeding so she does not attach much importance to it. She has occasional indigestion due to the 'rush over meals, as there is not much time after serving the family' . . . She has 24s. after paying 18s. rent, on which to feed, clothe and warm the family . . . She is usually on her feet for 12 hours a day but as she is breast feeding the twins she 'gets more rest' at present. In the evening she gets about two hours to herself when she does her mending, darning or knitting.

(3) Mrs B. of Paddington, 48, occupies two rooms in a four-storeyed house in a thickly populated district. Her husband is a scavenger. She has to go downstairs for her water and to empty away her dirty water. Three of her thirteen

[5] Margery Spring Rice, *op. cit.*

children died and she has had one miscarriage. Seven children now live at home. She gets up at 6.0 a.m. and goes to bed at 11.0 p.m.

The report continued:

Contraceptive advice seems practically non-existent. A few women in London, Rotherham and Devonshire speak of having been to the birth control clinics, but there are dozens of women in obvious need of such advice, either for procuring proper intervals between births, or to have no more children who, although they have been told by their doctor that this is necessary, are not instructed by him in scientific methods and do not go to a birth control clinic, even if there is one within reach.

Margery Spring Rice was confirming the experience of Marie Stopes, one of whose correspondents wrote appealing to her:

I want to bring no more babies into the world for their own little sakes. My husband is an ideal daddy. Since little Reggie came he has had no connections with me at all for he is afraid of my becoming pregnant again . . . and doctor, I will tell you something I dare tell no one else. I have found out my husband is 'abusing himself' . . . It is worrying me terribly because I am afraid to let him have anything to do with me. I am, though ignorant of such matters, sure he will do himself some harm.[6]

A particularly heart-rending letter to Marie from a wife of a labourer further illustrates the depth of despair suffered by women unable to avoid the chances of becoming pregnant against their wishes:

The third day after my confinement my husband came to my bedside and said it served me right that I was so bad, other women could prevent having children and so could I if I tried. Since then he has been very cruel to me because I will not submit to his embrace. He has often compelled me as he had done very, very many times before to submit with my back to him. He says 'If you won't let me at the front, I will at the back. I don't care which way it is as long as I get satisfaction.' Well, madam, this is very painful to me. Also I have wondered if it might be injurious. I feel that I hate my husband and cannot submit for

[6] Ruth Hall, ed. *Dear Dr Stopes: Sex in the 1920s*, André Deutsch, 1978.

fear of having any more children, and then be accused
unfaithfulness, but when all is said and done I am still his wif
and although I do not like just to be used for his pleasure and
then abused when I am pregnant, still unless I do submit, he
declares he will ask other women . . .[7]

As she spoke of these conditions at the Central Hall, Helena saw
dawning on the faces of her listeners 'the same rapt attention I had
observed as a novice speaker on the faces of the mothers of Wiltshire
and Dorset.'[8]

There were only three dissentients to Mrs Hubback's resolution
and it was sent to the Minister, Arthur Greenwood. It was the
beginning of the end of a ten-year fight most of which had been going
on while Helena was in China. As a result of this conference the
Ministry of Health conceded partial defeat by issuing three months
later Memorandum 153/MCW which allowed local authorities to give
instruction on birth control to women whose health would be injured
by further pregnancy.

Helena's next assignment was to speak for the newly formed
National Birth Control Council on 15 August 1930 at the Lambeth
Conference of Anglican bishops at which birth control was to be a
major issue for discussion. It was a considerable challenge which
Helena took up with typical confidence: 'I realised that, if not actually
hostile, there was nothing to encourage the belief that the Anglican
Church was sympathetic to the birth control movement, but I thought
I might as well try as I'd been asked to.'[9] She decided to use the same
technique, comparing two groups of women, which had proved
successful at the April conference in the Central Hall, Westminster.

The 1908 Lambeth Conference had 'viewed with alarm the growing
practice of artificial restriction of the family . . . as demoralising to
character and hostile to national welfare' and had condemned 'the
practice of resorting to artificial means for the avoidance or prevention
of childbearing'. But in 1920 the ecclesiastical members of the National Birth Rate Commission, of which Marie Stopes was a member, had supported family limitation, and Marie, hoping to push
home her advantage and claiming divine inspiration, sent a personal
message to every bishop attending the Lambeth Conference that year.

[7] Hall, ed., *op. cit.*
[8] Personal communication to the author—7.1.80.
[9] Personal communication to the author—7.1.80.

Their lordships were, alas, unimpressed and instead issued 'an emphatic warning against the use of unnatural means for the avoidance of conception, together with the grave dangers—physical, moral and religious, thereby incurred, and against the evils with which the extension of such use threatens the race', adding for good measure that 'the governing considerations of Christian marriage are the procreation of children and self control . . .'

By 1930 many Anglican bishops and clergy had modified their views. Aldous Huxley,[10] observing a general reduction in the size of clerical families, had already urged 'these gentlemen [to] bring themselves in time to preach what they already practise'. In due course Helena turned up at Church Hall, Westminster, to address the conference of over three hundred bishops from countries as far afield as Alaska, North China and Madras, including the then Archbishop of Canterbury, the Most Reverend C. G. Lang. They listened politely to this relatively young woman doctor. As Helena described the bishops:

> They seemed all to be white-haired, a mass of dear old gentlemen. One or two of them smiled when I told them they knew nothing about the people I was talking about, the women who had been my patients. These working-class mothers all had more children than they could afford. Sexual intercourse within marriage was the one factor they had never considered in the context of whether they wanted the children they had, whether they were able to support them, or if they could do anything about it. The women had come to the clinic because we had put notices on the door offering help. Each woman came in a state of wonderment. It was as if they had been told they could control the weather.
>
> I had no idea if the bishops would listen, but as I described the changes I had seen in these women, and as the pictures unfolded I saw their expressions getting more and more human, and the transformation of the corporate feeling. One or two would look up, and I realised, 'Yes, he's taken it in. He sees something new.' I don't know if you could call it luck, but it had worked.
>
> Personal communication to the author—28.7.80

[10] E. R. Norman, *Church and Society in England 1770–1970*, Clarendon Press, 1976.

After she had spoken there was a 'curious living silence', until one of the bishops asked if there was a danger in the technique, if it could hurt the mothers and what did the husbands think? Helena told them she couldn't say about the husbands, but that she had seen every woman twice and if there was any trouble she expected the woman would tell her on her next visit.

As was to be expected there was some determined opposition, but eventually the Conference passed Resolution 15 by 193 to 67 votes:

> Where there is a clearly felt moral obligation to limit or avoid parenthood, the method must be decided on Christian principles. The primary and obvious method is complete abstinence from intercourse (as far as may be necessary) in a life of discipline and self-control lived in the power of the Holy Spirit. Nevertheless in those cases where there is such a clearly felt moral obligation to limit or avoid parenthood, and where there is a morally sound reason for avoiding complete abstinence, the Conference agrees that other methods may be used, provided that this is done in the light of the same Christian principles. The Conference records its strong condemnation of the use of any methods of conception-control from motives of selfishness, luxury, or mere convenience.

The 1930 Lambeth Conference had thus admitted limited approval of the practice of contraception. It was a triumph for Helena and a striking success. The Conference has never gone back on this resolution nor criticised the National Birth Control Council (which later became the FPA), since that date. The 1958 Conference was to express firm approval of the principle of birth control and the 1968 Conference confirmed this.

The 1930 Conference went on to record its abhorrence of the 'sinful practice of abortion'. Although she had secured her major point, Helena was to hear the Conference finally reiterate that sexual intercourse between those who are not legally married was 'a grievous sin', and that the use of contraceptives did not remove the sin:

> . . . In view of widespread and increasing use of contraceptives among the unmarried and the extension of irregular unions, owing to the diminution of any fear of consequences, the Conference presses for legislation forbidding the exposure

for sale and the unrestricted advertisement of contraceptives and placing definite restrictions upon their purchase.[11]

This has not been achieved by legislation, although television companies have voluntarily restricted the advertising of contraceptives.

At the age of forty-one Helena was by now fully committed to a totally new career. Her work at the North Kensington Women's Welfare Centre was to be paid at the rate of £2 a weekly session, and she proposed to make up her income as a private gynaecologist specialising in birth control at a time when, undaunted, she recognised continuing medical antagonism to the subject and public apathy. Her sister Margaret by 1928 was a budding child psychiatrist and that year set up the Institute of Child Psychology in London. She had a private practice in Queen Anne Street and offered Helena the temporary use of her consulting room, until Helena and Peter rented their own rooms at 9 Weymouth Street.

Having now two fixed working points, Helena decided the time had come to leave Hounslow and look for a London house for the family, midway between Telford Road and Weymouth Street. Accordingly she got on her old friend the Number 6 bus, went to Maida Vale where she found an estate agent, and told him what she wanted. It was to be a large house in an unfashionable area which would therefore be easier to get—and pay for. It took a matter of hours to find 5 Randolph Crescent, a house which had belonged to the gynaecologist and obstetrician Aleck Bourne of St Mary's Hospital. Aleck Bourne was to become known for his bravery in terminating—then illegally—the pregnancy of a fourteen-year-old girl who had been the victim of rape. He then notified the police of his action and on 18 July 1938 was charged at the Central Criminal Court with 'unlawfully using an instrument with intent to procure miscarriage'. The defence was that it was 'for preserving the life of the mother'. He was found not guilty, and had fired the opening shot in his campaign for abortion law reform.

The new house was certainly large—four storeys—in a street where most of the other houses had been converted into flats. Peter got a building society loan, and paid the deposit on the head lease with the proceeds of the sale of the bungalow at Iltis Huk. The ground rent was

[11] *Lambeth Conference 1930*: Encyclical Letter from the Bishops with the Resolutions and Reports. Resolution 18.

£20 a year. Helena filled the house with the furniture which by then had been returned from China. She seems somehow to have been reasonably solvent, for she installed a French nurse for the boys, a cook, housemaid and butler, later to be replaced with a parlour maid, a staff roughly equivalent to the Lowndes Square ménage, except that no horses or grooms were included.

Helena threw herself heart and soul into her new life with her usual energy. She came increasingly in contact with voluntary crusaders in the emerging birth control movement, predominantly middle-class, politically motivated women concerned with women's welfare. By 1930 there were over thirty independently established birth control clinics in various parts of the country, all organised on a charitable basis and staffed by a combination of nurses, doctors and voluntary helpers. There were about five birth control societies, including Marie Stopes's Society for Constructive Birth Control (SCBC), Walworth's Society for the Provision of Birth Control Clinics (SPBCC) and the Birth Control Investigation Committee (BCIC) in which Mrs Spring Rice was interested. Then there was the Birth Control International Information Society (BCIIS) and the Workers Birth Control Group (WBCG).

Unlike Marie Stopes, who had designed her own cervical 'thimble' which fitted closely over the neck of the womb and was used with a quinine pessary, the other clinics advocated a spring-rim vaginal diaphragm fitted by a doctor and used with a spermicidal jelly, but some women failed to return for follow-up and little information was available on the clinical aspects of the methods. The Medical Committee of the National Birth Rate Commission had drawn attention in 1927 to the lack of scientific knowledge and the need for the collection of statistical data on the various contraceptive appliances used in different clinics. Accordingly the Birth Control Investigation Committee (BCIC) was formed that year (1927), with Sir Humphrey Rolleston as Chairman and Dr C. P. Blacker (later Hon. Secretary of the Eugenics Society) as joint Secretary with the Honourable Mrs Farrer.

After the April Conference at the Central Hall, Westminster, in 1930, a number of pioneers including Mrs Hugh Dalton, Eva Hubback and Mrs Gerda Guy, discussed with Margery Spring Rice the possibility of amalgamating these disparate voluntary bodies into one national organisation to correlate the research and centralise the work of providing birth control for the poor. Margery Spring Rice approached Lady Denman, a prominent social figure, and a number of exploratory meetings took place in London. Mrs Margaret Pyke, a woman of exceptional character and intelligence, asked Helena if she would serve on a preliminary committee.

Helena soon discovered that Marie Stopes was not to be included, one of the reasons being that Mrs Spring Rice, although she liked and respected Marie in some ways, thought her response to the Catholic opposition was unrealistic. After all, chaining her pamphlet, *Roman Catholic Methods of Birth Control*, to the Westminster Cathedral font as she had done was hardly likely to advance the cause. Other people had found her unreasonably didactic and autocratic; she might have been a splendid palaeontologist, but she had no medical authority. However, Helena refused to serve on the committee unless Marie was asked as well; this was agreed, providing Helena would 'manage' Marie. On 17 July 1930 a significant meeting took place at Lady Denman's house in Upper Grosvenor Street. At this gathering Marie Stopes and Ernest Thurtle, MP, proposed that 'the National Birth Control Council should be brought into being'. This became the National Birth Control Association (NBCA) in 1931 and was the forerunner of the FPA which was established in 1939. Mrs Margaret Pyke, 'a genius at this sort of thing' as Helena appropriately called her, became the first Secretary of the NBCC for derisory pay, Lady Denman the Chairman, and Sir Thomas (later Lord) Horder, the eminent physician, its first President, a sign of changing medical opinion. Lord Horder remained President until his death twenty-five years later.

Helena had wanted Marie Stopes to be a member of the NBCA Executive Committee, believing her views were important, but from the beginning, as others had foreseen, she showed herself an uncooperative member. Dr Evelyn Fisher, a general practitioner who joined the staff of Marie's clinic to help with medical problems in 1931 and liked and admired Marie Stopes for her compassion, knew her also as 'a very determined woman who wasn't going to be told how to do things by anybody'. As Marie had put it, 'I'm not the Cabin Boy in this movement. I'm the Admiral.' This mentality destroyed the harmony of the NBCA Executive Committee meetings, whose members listened politely in silence to Marie before Margaret Pyke moved to the next item on the agenda. Realising she could not influence the other members, Marie resigned from the Executive in 1933 to battle on alone in her Constructive Birth Control Society.

On the day Marie left, Helena drove her home in her car. 'She was in a blazing rage,' according to Helena, and said Helena was the only member of the NBCA in whom she had any confidence. 'Dr Wright,' she asked Helena, 'could you find me a woman doctor who will run my birth control clinic in my way and under my instructions?' to which Helena could only reply, 'Dr Stopes, such a woman does not exist.'

Helena, as Chairman of the Medical Sub-Committee of the NBCC, served on the Executive Committee with five prominent women, Mary Stocks, Eva Hubback, Margery Spring Rice, Marie Stopes and Margaret Pyke. Mary Stocks and Mrs Hugh Dalton were on the Public Relations Sub-Committee. Helena greatly admired Eva Hubback who was, according to Helena, 'tall and Junoesque with a brown velvet voice. It could resound and echo; it could be gentle, or it could bite very effectively.' Eva for her part envied Helena's 'robustness'. Eva could interpret Helena's ideas for the benefit of the lay committee:

> She never talked nonsense, never interrupted, but everyone listened to her if she had something new to say. She was full of ideas and very businesslike, as well as being practical and courageous. I would say to her, 'Now, Eva, you explain in *your* words what *I'm* saying medically. They'll understand if you tell it them your way.'
>
> Personal communication to the author—28.1.80

Another thing about Eva that appealed to Helena was that she 'had the privilege of being totally Jewish, while I have the privilege of being only *half* Jewish and I'm not even certain about that'.

Eva was also good at raising money, one of the major functions of the lay committee and a recurring problem in spite of Lady Denman's generous support, without which, as Margaret Pyke has said, the NBCA could not have kept going. In 1931 its status was changed with its acceptance by the Charity Commissioners. The lay committee's task in addition to money-raising now involved reorganisation and the extension of its work throughout the country, in creating more clinics and in maintaining standards.

As Chairman for five years of the Medical Sub-Committee on which her friend and neighbour Dr Joan Malleson also served, Helena guided the lay committee past important milestones. Together she and Joan Malleson made birth control both respectable and available. Ahead of its time in realising the importance of quality control, the

NBCA issued in 1934 an *Approved List of Proprietary Contraceptives*. There was then no Committee on the Safety of Medicines as there is now and no watchdog either on manufacturers. The NBCA instigated, on Helena's insistence, rigorous testing of spermicides, rubber condoms and caps. Every product had to be safe *and* effective. There had been differences of opinion on the merits of vaginal or cervical caps. Opinion was also divided on the efficacy of different spermicides. Maries Stopes favoured cocoa-butter pessaries with chinosol, and the Society for the Provision of Birth Control Clinics favoured quinine with a gelatine base. These products were carefully tested for their sperm-killing properties and the recommended list sent by the NBCA to all voluntary clinics and to any doctor who applied.

On Dr C. P. Blacker's initiative a survey was instigated into the chemical effects of products which had been introduced without previous testing. Dr John Baker in Oxford was asked to investigate possible spermicides. His colleagues disapproved. 'Who's interested in sperms?' was his own initial reaction, but his work resulted in the discovery, in 1936, of the spermicidal preparation containing phenyl-mercuric acetate which was christened Volpar (Voluntary Parenthood) which is still available as paste, gels and foaming tablets. The NBCA made a grievous mistake in not cashing in on what should have been a considerable financial asset. By buying the ingredients wholesale, manufacturing themselves and selling directly to patients the NBCA made £200 a month, but then gave sole distribution rights of Volpar to a commercial firm, British Drug Houses, specifying only a reasonable profit. 'Ladies, ladies,' said the BDH Marketing Manager, 'you are throwing away a fortune.'

However, the ladies refused to listen to financial reason and did not want commercial involvement. Helena later expressed her regret to me: 'We were sentimental idealists. We should have noticed what Sweden was doing when their leader, Mrs Elise Ottesen-Jensen, realised that the Swedish Family Planning organisation could support itself on the sales of proprietary spermicides.' The NBCA could have done with the cash sales. In 1931 its income was just over £600 which had to cover Mrs Pyke's salary of £200 per annum.

Meanwhile Helena had brought to the Telford Road Clinic all the organising ability she showed at the NBCA. She had elaborated a training syllabus for prospective specialists in birth control involving three sessions, after which candidates would be examined by one of the training doctors, including an oral review. Volunteers were enlisted from among the patients and rewarded by a cup of tea and a bun in return for their activities as a human model. Every successful candidate received a numbered certificate of competence, each personally signed by Helena.

Slowly she had begun to involve the reluctant and indifferent members of the medical profession. The British Postgraduate Medical School at Hammersmith was the first medical school in Britain to provide lectures on contraception. They were given by Helena in 1936. She described the appropriate methods and the necessary organisation and equipment of clinics. The failure rate of contraception varied from 1 per cent to 6 per cent, but statistical assessment had proved difficult because not all women returned for follow-up. But, she said, this was improving. In the early years at Telford Road among 1,000 women, 60 per cent failed to return after the first visit. Two to three years later 40 per cent of another 1,000 women failed to return. At the time she was speaking only 10 per cent of the latest 1,000 women had not reported after the first visit. The results tallied, she said, 'rather surprisingly' with those in her private practice. She touched finally on the psychological aspect, describing it as 'all-pervading in the whole theme, but always individual in solution'. She aptly summed up: 'No method will be used continuously which annoys either partner.'

[9]

Spreading the Message

The field of psychosexual counselling at the Telford Road clinic was covered by Dr Joan Malleson, but in her own consulting room at 9 Weymouth Street Helena's time was her own. There she was free to deal with the sexual problems which she uncovered in patients who had come primarily for contraceptive advice, but who often as they left her consulting room would turn at the door and say shyly, 'And another thing, doctor . . .' As she told me:

> I soon realised how low was the level of sexual success among these women. I had come back from China where the subject of sex was never discussed to find Marie Stopes beginning to stir up the hidden depths of repressed female sexuality. I estimated that at least fifty per cent of married women in my practice failed to achieve sexual satisfaction. I conceived it to be part of my professional responsibility to deal with a situation which was spoiling the lives of my patients, becoming an unnecessary tragedy, compelling attention. It was as if they wanted to knit, but didn't know how to hold the needles.
>
> Personal communication to the author—31.7.81

Helena found this side of her work expanded increasingly and she was interested and active in psychosexual therapy long before this had become a specialty in its own right. She believed she was successful here because she was a woman and that women spoke freely to her because her matter-of-fact, prosaic approach spared them the embarrassment which discussion of sexual matters might induce in consultation with men.

In fact more than one woman who had been her patient has said that Helena did not give her the particular feeling of being treated by a woman. It is said that one clinic patient thought she had been seen by a man doctor. She did not speak to patients as one woman to another, but as doctor to patient in the way a man might speak dispassionately

about female ailments. As one woman said, there was nothing feminine about the businesslike, small, plainly dressed, rather squat
woman with short hair and bright eyes behind pince-nez glasses. Her
male colleagues do not seem to have thought of her as being particularly feminine either, rather the reverse. Even women who loved Helena
either as friends or as patients have said they were intimidated by her
at times. One of her friends, Mrs Joan Rettie, who worked with her
first at Telford Road and later in the International Planned Parenthood Federation, has said that although Helena never intended to
hurt, she did not always understand that others might not think or
react as she did herself, looking at problems usually through her own
eyes.

Ahead of her time once again, Helena was among the first sex
therapists in Britain, though that is not how she would have described
herself. She came to believe that the sexual education of women was
one of modern society's major innovations, comparable with the
improvement in the general education of women and equal to the
realisation that women were as entitled to general education as men.
Her technique differed from those which modern sex therapists have
evolved, but she taught women to achieve freedom from fear—fear of
sex, fear of taboos, fear of public opinion, with freedom to make their
own choice. She was approachable and she had endless time. She
would talk to any woman as long as she wished, arguing that the next
appointment could always wait.

Unlike later sex therapists and the marriage counsellors of her own
generation, Helena did not see both husbands and wives together. If a
woman's sexual partner wanted Helena's advice he could ring up and
make his own appointment and many did, but not as a rule for a
tripartite consultation. It amused her to tell the tale of a husband who
came to see her with his wife's knowledge, to discuss where his sexual
approach to his wife was at fault. As he was leaving her consulting
room he turned to Helena and said rather timidly, 'Do you think you
could get her to take off her nightdress?' In a way, it was a joke against
herself and her emphasis on the importance of touch. As I have said,
her tendency was to see a problem only from the feminine angle, or
perhaps from her own personal prejudice.

It is important to remember the almost unbelievable level of public
ignorance in Helena's day and the total inability of large sections of the
population to discuss anything related to genital function. Helena
used to start off her consultation about sexual anxieties with a

physiology lesson. She had a drawing of a nude given her by her friend
the artist Eric Gill above the examination couch, showing the penis
from the lateral view. After physiology she could deal with anatomy.
The preliminaries consisted of a description of the special senses, and
their individual triggers and the individual nerve supply. As an
example, taking sight, in which the optic nerve is involved, she would
say, 'Here the trigger is light.' The patient was then instructed to work
out the similarity of function and comparable trigger with hearing
—the answer being 'noise' or 'sound'.

It was then time to demonstrate the function of sensory nerves in
the skin. With a light probe Helena would touch the girl's inner thigh,
then her pubic hair and lastly the clitoris. She would get out a mirror
and let the girl see what the small pink object looked like, which gave
such a specific reaction to touch. The lesson ended with a dissertation
on rhythmic friction—the all-important trigger with its specific individual pattern for each woman. Helena would tell the girl or woman
that she must teach her partner her own rhythm and make it clear that
adjustment must be made for the fact that, unlike a woman's, the
male's sexual impulse is an instinctive action which achieves a climax
independently of individual variation. Women, Helena would explain, respond to men if they are in sympathy with them, as they
respond to different musical instruments.

Helena had a different technique for women who had had multiple
partners—a situation probably less common in her day than in ours,
but one which she was prepared to encourage. She loved lovers, and
told one reporter who came to interview her in her old age, in her
matter-of-fact way, 'You have eyes, you have ears, and you have a
lover.' Helena would go to considerable lengths to help lovers in a
predicament, making only one important provision: the stability of a
good marriage should not be prejudiced.

She had worked out for herself how to deal with the ever-present
opposition of the Catholic Church, and where Marie Stopes regarded
the Catholics as implacable enemies, Helena evolved a method which
entailed some compromise on the part of a Catholic patient who came
for contraceptive advice. Again this is not unusual today, but in the
Thirties and Forties the obstacles were considerably greater. Helena
gave her patients advice which was intended to maintain and not
imperil a Catholic patient's religious convictions. She had herself been
influenced by her mother's religion—that of the Church of England
—and she was the daughter of a Jewish father who ultimately became

a Catholic, after his own mother, Rosa, had embraced the Catholic faith.

When asked by a Catholic patient, 'But what will the priest say about all this?' Helena would then reply, 'Well, it's the priest we must be sorry for. It is he who is trying to prevent you from thinking out a problem for yourself. You have seen a little of the truth. You are not a child to be dictated to. It is for you to decide what you tell your priest. No Protestant would forgo the right of personal judgement, but this is not sufficient cause for you to change your religion.' This would not have needed saying nowadays, when compromise is easier to establish and relations between priest and penitent are more elastic.

Another doctrinal conflict could arise in the case of women who came to Helena with a problem of infertility. The couple wanted children and in order to establish their failure to become parents when there seemed no reason for the woman's inability to conceive, it was necessary to examine the seminal fluid. For this test semen is collected by masturbation, something which the Catholic Church has regarded as sinful, though more so in Helena's day than in ours. It was Helena's practice to ask to see the confessor of a Catholic woman in this predicament. She would never call a priest 'Father'. 'Now, Mr So-and-So,' she would say, 'Mrs X wants to have a baby who will, if I am successful in helping her, become a member of the Catholic Church. It is in the interests of your Church that you should allow me to do this test.' The battle was not even joined before Helena had won it for her patient.

Where sex was concerned Helena taught her patients in the light of her own experience; their difficulties had been her own problems. Marriage to another virgin, five years her junior, had not been easy. She frankly described to me her own sexual initiation at the age of thirty:

> In order to become a father a male cannot help experiencing the highest level of local physical pleasure; that's what he thinks about, not about being a father. This accounts for all the horrors of their cruelty, their selfishness . . . Peter being the kind, kind man he was, and having been brought up so far away from this idea, never thought in the least about it—I had to tell him. 'Peter,' I said, 'I find this a bore.' It wasn't boring to him. He had his orgasm all right. 'Oh dear,' he said. 'I'm so sorry,' as if he'd broken a teacup.

. . . I had learnt about the hymen from textbooks—not from the gynaecologists who should have taught us as students—they would never discuss that sort of thing. I stretched it myself, first with one finger, then two, until I could get three in. First intercourse wasn't painful, but everything felt dead. I didn't want to wound Peter, but I thought to myself, 'There must be some other way of doing this.'

Personal communication to the author—3.2.81

She had turned to the *Kama Sutra*, read all six volumes of Havelock Ellis's *Studies in the Psychology of Sex* (1896), and *Die Homosexualität* (1914) by Magnus Hirschfeld, the German authority on sexual studies. She then set about applying the lessons in her own sex life. 'Peter was endlessly kind and it was impossible to offend him. I said to him, "Now we're going to experiment," and we did.'

Later she was to read Theodore van de Velde's *Ideal Marriage: Its Physiology and Technique* (1926). She regarded this book by the Dutch gynaecologist as 'of the greatest value to the medical profession' and acknowledged her debt to the author in the preface to the first book she herself wrote for the benefit of her own patients when she realised their general sexual ignorance, *The Sex Factor in Marriage* (1930). Of van de Velde it has been said that he taught a generation of men and women to copulate, a generation raised on the concept that sex was inherently evil. They were thus untrained in the art of sexual responsiveness between a reciprocally functioning couple. Originally written in Dutch and German 'for doctors and married men', the book was translated into English in 1928. A revised edition was still in print in paperback fifty years later.

In writing his comprehensive manual on sexual intercourse, van de Velde left virtually nothing to the imagination and advocated both fellatio and cunnilingus. While concentrating on the cultivation of the technique of eroticism, he aimed at 'an entirely scientific tone . . . free from superfluous pedantry'. This gave his work a more clinical slant than Helena's. Moreover his attitude was primarily oriented towards the man. While Helena wrote in *The Sex Factor in Marriage*, 'The wife who means to have a happy sex life should decide with all her strength that she *wants* her body to feel all the sensation of sex with the greatest possible vividness,' van de Velde had written in *Ideal Marriage*, 'The wife must be *taught* not only how to behave in coitus, but above all how and what to feel in this unique act.' The man should be the initiator, the woman the willing pupil. While Helena evidently believed the woman should control the timing of coitus, she still thought with Havelock Ellis and van de Velde that the woman's sexual desire should be orchestrated by the man, who must learn to play the tune his partner liked, but it was his job to awaken her sexuality. Marie Stopes maintained on the contrary that sexual intercourse should depend on the woman's biological rhythm in which peaks of desire coincide with ovulation and the period immediately preceding the onset of menstruation when the pelvic organs are congested. According to Marie a good sexual partner should learn to adapt to this female rhythm. Unlike Marie Stopes, Helena held the view shared with Havelock Ellis that women may not realise they want sexual intercourse until it is offered. Where they all three agreed was on the importance of wooing on the part of the man.

In spite of its success elsewhere, *Ideal Marriage* was suppressed in Germany when Hitler came to power. Three years earlier Helen's publishers had entertained doubts that *The Sex Factor in Marriage* might be suppressed in England, and took the precaution of burying two copies of the manuscript, one in France and the other in England, for fear the police would confiscate all the copies on publication. No doubt with these fears in mind, they had shrewdly included a 'frank' introduction by a Nonconformist parson, the Reverend Herbert Gray, a friend of Helena's, who admitted to feelings of guilt that the Church did not provide for those for whom it performed the sacrament of marriage a 'clear and healthy knowledge of the terms on which success in marriage can be attained'. As if this were not enough to bestow ecclesiastical blessing on the book, the dust cover carried an extract from a speech delivered to the London Diocesan Council for Rescue Work at the Mansion House on 4 April 1930 by the same Archbishop of Canterbury, Dr Lang, who was later that year to hear Helena address the Lambeth Conference.

> I would rather have all the risks which come from a free discussion of sex than the great risks we run by a conspiracy of silence . . . We want to liberate the sex impulse from the impression that it is always to be surrounded by negative warnings and restraints, and to place it in its rightful place among the great creative and formative things.

The Sex Factor in Marriage is a beginner's guide to sexual intercourse which Helena intended 'for those who are, or are about to be married'. It was to become a best-seller with sales of over a million and was translated into Greek, Dutch, Swedish and Norwegian. It contains 'explicit instructions on the art of love-making within marriage'.

> The false idea that intercourse undertaken for a reproductive purpose is more meritorious than intercourse performed purely as an expression of love is dying. It never had any foundation in reason or science . . . As long as we have bodies . . . every healthy person will continue to have sex needs . . . A successful and satisfactory sex relation is within the reach of every married couple who are willing to take the trouble about it.

Description of the male and female reproductive organs and their functions emphasised the nature and importance of the clitoris, 'whose sole purpose is to produce sensation'. In Helena's telling phraseology, 'Nearly all women find vaginal sensation through, as it were, the gateway of clitoris sensation.'

Helena compared the attitude to sex among primitive peoples with that in England which she considered 'unhealthy, ignorant and thoroughly unsatisfactory'. Eastern people, she averred, 'never leave a knowledge of sex to chance . . . It is considered a deep and social disgrace if a man marries and proves himself incapable of rousing and satisfying his wife's physical nature.' She attributed the unsatisfactory state of affairs in her own country to ignorance of the fundamental difference between male and female response to sex stimulation, men being quicker to arouse and quicker to satisfy. Women require longer and persistent clitoral stimulation, by various techniques and in a number of possible positions, which husbands might fail to appreciate.

Fifty years later these views are universally accepted, if not always applied, but in the Thirties they were considered unmentionable by the vast majority, many of whom had not even heard of the clitoris. Indeed, one of Helena's readers, a herdsman, wrote to say that he had taken his fiancée up into the heather to try to locate her clitoris, but concluded that she had not got one.

Besides the numerous women she helped, many of Helena's admirers were men. Among those who expressed their appreciation, a reader of *The Sex Factor in Marriage* wrote from Massachusetts in 1936 to say that it had changed his life and he wished he and his wife could have read it earlier. A South African who used the book in the youth centre he ran wrote in 1957 to say he was glad Helena had made it clear that sexual activity could be continued into later years. At the age of seventy-two with a wife six years his junior, he could endorse Helena's views. Then there was the bachelor clergyman who found it helpful in preparing his parishioners in 'the important sex aspects of marriage'. Two of his flock had been brought up in an orphanage and remained abstinent after marriage, as they had been threatened in youth with hellfire if they were not. When he met them several years later the wife thanked him—'It should really be you,' he wrote to Helena—as they had had a normal, happy life as a result of his advice.

Of course she also had her critics—many of them men. Among the earlier ones was Eric Gill, the erotic artist and sculptor known as 'the Married Monk', a nickname given to him for his intense attempts to fuse the erotic and the divine. A man of strong erotic feelings embedded in the spiritual life, he was converted to Catholicism after marriage and later became a Dominican Tertiary. His 'Ariel', the genitalia suitably diminished on the BBC Governors' orders, still presides over Broadcasting House. Gill became a close friend and helped Helena with her own painting at which she was more than a talented amateur.

Gill had done the frieze in the sitting-room of Tom Hill's London house, and he and Helena often met in Tom's country house. She remembered Gill's eccentric clothes, the brown belted monk's habit.

All artists are self-centred, so he wasn't interested in my work —not very, but I was interested in him. He had no scientific side to him, and our arguments were mainly about Catholicism, virgin birth, the supremacy of the Pope. His arguments were emotionally based and I thought Eric failed centrally in logic. We agreed as friends that we would never agree.

Personal communication to the author—31.7.80

From his house, Pigotts, near High Wycombe Gill wrote to Helena on 31 January 1933:

Dear Dr Wright,

I hope you will have a pleasant journey to the South of France and a good time there. This is to say I hope we'll have opportunity soon after your return to continue our discussion. Meanwhile here are a few notes for consideration. It seems to me you have a rather exclusively hospital nurse point of view. Perhaps this is inevitable. You don't seem to see or appreciate the essentially Rabelaisian quality of life. You're romantic. You don't sufficiently appreciate the difference between the psychology of the sex act in men and women.

You don't appreciate that sex act with contraception is the same as homosexuality. You don't seem to be aware that the control of *contraception by the woman* is essentially Matriarchy. If you are aware of this you don't say so. (Ask Mussolini!) Matriarchy is the (probably) inevitable conclusion of our Industrialised Commercialism. The two things (Industrialised Commercialism and Birth Control by the woman) are complementary. You are entitled to believe in and work for a matriarchal state. Men are equally entitled to resist it.

I believe in birth control by the man by means of:

(1) Karetza.
(2) Abstinence from intercourse.
(3) Withdrawal before ejaculation.
(4) French letters.

I don't think 3 and 4 are good. I don't think abstinence from orgasm is necessarily a bad thing. It depends on the state of mind and states of mind can be cultivated. (Anyway there's no point in ejaculating seed into a woman who doesn't welcome it—they can jolly well go without, if they don't want our spunk they needn't have it.)

Let us talk about Matriarchy next time—and Commercialism.

Yours sincerely,

Eric Gill

There is no record of Helena's reply but on 22 February 1933 Gill wrote to thank her for writing 'at such length'. It is safe to assume she was stung by his imputing to her a hospital nurse's point of view.

I fear we have not discovered a common language. Unbridgeable chasms seem to yawn between us. Still, I like trying to find or make bridges so I hope we shall continue.

Hospital nurses. Yes I've known a good few, but the point is not that hospital nurses hold such and such views, but that such and such views are appropriate to hospital nurses . . . I don't understand your remark about my 'lack of technical knowledge'. However you will enlighten me and I shall gladly learn . . .

Yours sincerely,
Eric Gill

Another man, much more directly and more acutely involved, presumably because of his wife's indoctrination by Helena in some —unspecified—aspect of her philosophy, wrote on 24 July 1930:

Dear Madam,

I feel I must write and tell you of the awful ruption you have caused in a decent man's home. You are slowly but surely separating a man and wife and robbing two fine little boys of the sight of their father and I am sure it will harm them . . . For a lady to tell any wife that she can do such a thing in her married life and all through life and that the husband has no choice in the matter at all I never thought that there was a Christian alive like it. Won't you write me and say you never said this and my wife will never see you again I feel sure.

Yours Very Broken Hearted.

PS   It will take years for me to think of my wife in the old way again.

Writing came easily to Helena, and spurred on by the success of *The Sex Factor in Marriage* she moved on to the sex education of the adolescent. She had met a group of public school boys from Marlborough College who found her uninhibited conversation instructive, and begged for more. She took them on a picnic in Savernake Forest and then went to see their headmaster, George Turner. As a result in 1932 she produced *What is Sex? An Outline for Young People*. It was published in America by The Vanguard Press under the title *The Story of Sex* (1932). Helena had with some difficulty persuaded George Turner to write the introduction, thus making a controversial subject educationally acceptable. Mr Turner admired Helena, but was said to be frightened by her. Not so the boys; they thoroughly enjoyed her refreshing attitude to sex, which at least one master thought too liberal, and a few boys continued the discussions with her in London in the holidays on their own initiative.

Archbishop Lang's quotation appeared once again on the dust cover of *What is Sex?* Rather more than half the book dealt with sex in plants and animals and this was followed by an account of the reproductive biology of human beings. It went on to the psychology of both sexes, before and after marriage. Helena condemned the practice of prostitution, pointed out the risks and dangers of genital infection and finally was back on the subject of self-stimulation which she classified among the activities which 'growing young people should be prepared to leave . . . behind as they become more and more capable of taking part in the real things of life'.

The book was a bonus for parents and teachers who found talking freely to the young embarrassing, but reckoned it their duty to give them the facts. Its success can be gauged by the fact that it was still in print in 1947, although by then dated, especially in respect of the alleged dangers and need for medical treatment of masturbation if allowed to become a fixed habit. Helena hoped young people of the future would ultimately harness these instincts in 'enough outlets of energy in mental and physical occupations . . . until they are able to earn their own livings, and then they will marry one another and each . . . will go on working, if necessary, so that the financial burdens of marriage can be supported by both instead of one'.

Helena could not forbear to note that the mental and spiritual dissatisfaction resulting from a union concerned only with the physical aspect is generally felt more keenly by the woman. 'To the normal feminine nature, physical love for a man is so intimately bound up with the natural desire for a home and constant companionship, that more often than not, a temporary sex adventure is more potent in creating pain than in conferring relief.'

It was perhaps unfortunate, in view of its eventual universal acceptance, that Helena saw no future at this stage in the use of the word 'contraception', regarding it as too cumbersome, 'although its meaning is exactly what we want it is hopeless to expect that . . . it will ever attain popular usage'. She preferred the term 'family spacing' to 'birth control', a phrase coined by Margaret Sanger. When she was asked by Cassell, the publishers, to write a book on the subject Helena chose as her title *Birth Control: Advice on Family Spacing and Healthy Sex Life* (1935). It originally cost 6d. and, by 1948, 7s.6d. For some reason Helena had to be nagged by Cassell to write this book for their Health Handbook series. She had not herself conceived the notion that the general public required educating on the technical aspects of birth control, but when finally persuaded to fill this gap she sat down there and then and completed the exercise in one night without sleep. By breakfast time it was finished, over 20,000 words. The book covered the disadvantages of the methods which were currently in use—*coitus interruptus*; *coitus reservatus* in which ejaculation does not occur; the rhythm method sanctioned by the Catholic Church; abstinence and abortion; and then described the preferred barrier methods. These were still the sheath and the varieties of cap used in combination with spermicides, but Helena added, for the benefit of women who lived in rural areas without access to a clinic, an account of the age-old method, a home-made device consisting of a ball of cotton wool soaked in dilute vinegar on a string.

It was now (1935) that Helena first referred to extramarital sexual intercourse as socially permissible but, surprisingly in view of later criticism, this apparently went unchallenged at the time. In rejecting the objection to contraception on moral grounds, Helena maintained that there could be no danger to society from

> . . . a growing class of thoughtful people who seriously hold the view that sexual intercourse outside marriage is a good and healthy practice if it is reasonably managed . . . Society should recognise the fundamental rights of every responsible individual to liberty of private action as long as such action remains private.

She was already applying this principle in her private life.

Helena Wright will probably be best remembered for *The Sex Factor in Marriage*, but the importance of the Cassell booklet should not be ignored. In it she urged the Ministry of Health to withdraw all restrictions on contraceptive services by local authorities, and to set up birth control clinics throughout the country. It was time, she thought, for the government to take over the birth control services.

A ban had been imposed in 1924 which specifically forbade Welfare Centres from giving contraceptive advice in any circumstances. This ban had subsequently been partially lifted following pressure by feminist bodies. Margaret Pyke as Secretary of the newly formed NBCC had personally been able to interview the Minister of Health and this resulted in the now famous memorandum 153/MCW of July 1930, which as already noted on page 139 conceded that *married women whose health would be injured by further pregnancy* (my italics) could henceforth be given birth control instruction by local authorities. This was far from an enforcement on the authorities. On the contrary, the relevant document was typewritten, it was not printed as an official publication, and emerged by stealth in semi-secrecy. It was not issued to the press or to local authorities generally, but Marie Stopes printed a copy in *Birth Control News*. The following year as the result of pressure by the NBCA it was officially reprinted and fully circulated to local authorities, but with further 'clarification' aimed at curbing the enthusiasm of some authorities. Thirty-five out of four hundred and nine were by then providing some birth control services.

There was moreover ambiguity over the financial provision for the service. But by 1934, the year before *Birth Control* was published, the Ministry of Health did extend the powers of local authorities by allowing them to provide birth control for married women with conditions other than gynaecological ones. These now included tuberculosis and other chronic illnesses which could render pregnancy dangerous to health. It was an advance, but those who disapproved continued to evade their responsibilities. The town clerk would say that advice was available if asked for; the medical officer of health would maintain that his staff had not been asked to provide it.

Helena included a copy of a clarifying Ministry memorandum in the appendix to *Birth Control*. She devoted a chapter to the urgency of a situation officially recognised by the Minister of Health, but which few local authorities had troubled to implement. The book also publicised the extended facilities offered by the FPA and urged readers to lobby parliamentary candidates in support of measures authorising the Ministry of Health to organise birth control clinics on a national scale, and to pressurise medical officers of health. 'Whether he approves or not he has to carry out the wishes of the Council or resign his office,' wrote Helena.

Many family doctors, while limiting their own families, still disapproved of giving contraceptive advice for others. Helena told her readers that there was

---

(above right) *New Delhi, 1959. Sixth International Conference, International Planned Parenthood Federation, at which Helena (left) was elected Vice President of the IPPF. Dr Margaret Jackson (centre), UK, and Professor V. R. Khanolkar (right), Director, Indian Cancer Research Centre, Bombay, reported on the testing of contraceptives.*

(right) *Brighton, 1973. Twenty-first Anniversary Conference of the International Planned Parenthood Federation, when one of three Founders' Awards was named after Helena Wright. Far left another award winner, Lady Rama Rao (India). Helena is seated between Dr Siva Chinnatamby (Ceylon) and Professor Karl-Heinz Mehlan (Rostock), with Professor Hans Harmsen (Hamburg) behind her. 'We realised the world was the limit of the future.' Photograph Pic Photos.*

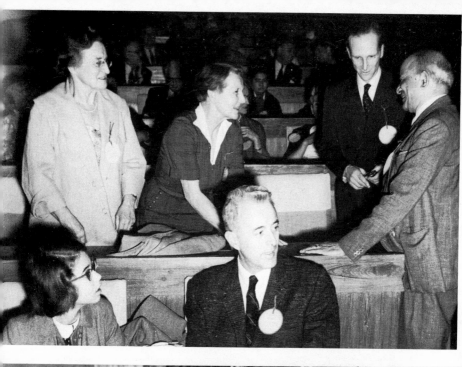

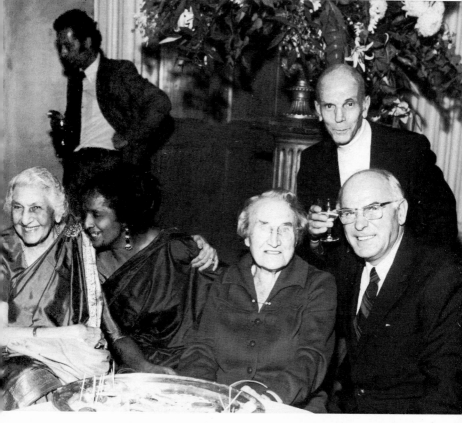

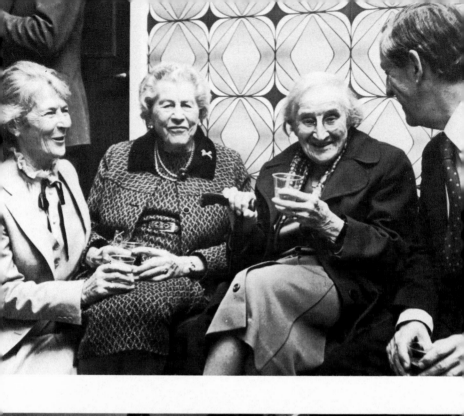
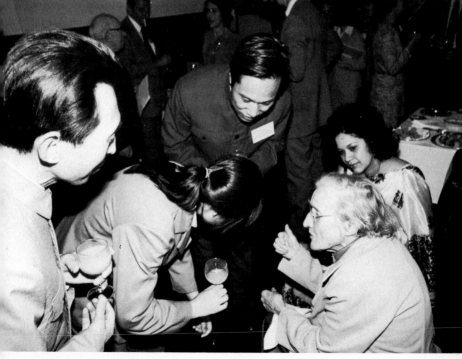

. . . nothing to prevent every woman . . . from going to her own family doctor and demanding help . . . as soon as they understand that their patients are serious in their desire for contraceptive instruction the doctors will obtain the necessary special training and will prepare themselves to begin the work . . .

She and the other pioneers had set the ball rolling, but success was not to come until the middle Fifties.

By then Helena had written her only book specifically for the medical profession, *Contraceptive Technique: A Handbook for Medical Practitioners and Senior Students*, with the assistance of H. Beric Wright, MB, BS (Lond.), (1951). The book dealt with the barrier methods currently used with a chemical spermicide, the sheath for men and the cap for women. The Pill had not arrived in the United Kingdom, but she made passing reference to the forerunner of the intra-uterine device, the wishbone pessary, a metal Y-shaped device which she condemned as being in no sense a contraceptive and which carried, she believed, a risk of infection. She referred also to the Gräfenberg Ring, a tightly coiled spring of silver or gold for insertion into the uterine cavity. She had met Dr Gräfenberg, its inventor, in Berlin on her way back from China. When publicising his device in England, Dr Gräfenberg had not mentioned the possibility of his ring falling out without the woman's knowledge. When this happened to one of her patients while in the bath, Helena had taken the next plane to Berlin to find out the truth and to give Dr Gräfenberg a piece of her mind. In *Contraceptive Technique* she observed that in occasional cases pregnancy had occurred in spite of the ring being in position. In a number of cases the ring had fallen out without the patient's knowledge, and she therefore considered its unreliability rendered it obsolete.

(above left) *1980. Honoured guest at the celebrations to mark the move of the Margaret Pyke Centre to the Soho Hospital for Women. Left to right Lady Medawar, Lady Limerick, Helena and Dr David Pyke.*
Photograph Cyril Bernard.

(left) *House of Commons, 11 May 1981. Reception for the delegation from the China Family Planning Association. Secretary General Mr Wang Liancheng (centre) and interpreter Ms Qiao Xinjian talking to Helena who had not forgotten her Mandarin. Dr Pramilla Senanayake, Medical Director of the IPPF, is behind Helena.*
Courtesy IPPF and Jeremy Hamand.

More importantly, in this book Helena showed herself a propagandist. When describing the work of the FPA she noted that there were at the date of publication of *Contraceptive Technique* only twelve contraceptive clinics qualified to teach doctors and medical students, while the attitude of the Ministry of Health remained unsatisfactory. The 1946 National Health Service Act had made no mention whatsoever of family planning, and the Ministry of Health was anxious to avoid interfering in this politically sensitive field. Local councils were unwilling to accept responsibility for birth control under the newly formed, so-called comprehensive National Health Service. So the FPA continued to run its clinics at a financial disadvantage. The press exerted a virtual ban on publicity amounting to a conspiracy of silence, and as late as 1950 the BBC would not allow a broadcast appeal for the FPA. Pioneers such as Mary Stocks were insulted in public and, apart from a few enthusiasts, the official support of the professional gynaecological hierarchy was still lacking.

This obstructive attitude lasted into the 1950s with continuing opposition from many members of the medical and gynaecological hierarchy. In 1947 the Dean of Guy's had criticised the President of the Students' Union for inviting Helena to speak in the medical school. Other medical school teachers were also critical, but the students persisted. In the late 1930s a brave and foresighted young gynaecological registrar, W. C. W. Nixon, had asked if he might bring groups of five or six students from neighbouring St Mary's Hospital to Helena's clinic in Telford Road for lectures and demonstrations. Mrs Spring Rice decided they could not refuse to allow this but the students came under cover of darkness as they could not be seen coming to a birth control clinic in daylight. Later, as Professor of Gynaecology at University College Hospital, Professor Nixon was to lead the way by organising the first London family planning clinic in the out-patient department of a London teaching hospital.

A significant change in the public's attitude, amounting to a dramatic reversal of its former indifference to the birth control movement, came about in 1955, when within a few months contraception suddenly became publicly acceptable. This was due to the political courage and independence of mind of Iain Macleod, the Minister of Health. Lady Monckton, wife of Sir Walter Monckton, had recently joined the executive committee of the FPA and she invited Mr Macleod, a family friend, to lunch with Margaret Pyke the Chairman of the Association. When he learnt from Margaret Pyke of the difficulties the FPA was experiencing in gaining recognition, Iain Macleod asked her why she did not invite him to visit the headquarters. As a result he made an official visit with full-scale publicity on 29 November 1955 to celebrate the Silver Jubilee of the FPA. He also went to the Telford Road clinic, agreed to publication of his photograph, and gave a statement to the press.

In his speech he regretted that government responsibility for advising married women about contraception was not more widely known, adding, 'The dangers of going too slowly are worse than the dangers of going too fast.' This was the focal point for the publicity in the press and on television which followed. Public opinion changed almost overnight. 'The speed was the most fascinating social change I have ever seen,' according to Dr David Pyke, Margaret Pyke's son.[1] After Iain Macleod's visit only one Minister of Health, Enoch Powell, asked for a ban on publicity during an official visit to the FPA.

News of Helena's practice continued to spread by word of mouth from patient to patient, friend to friend and in the late Forties women began asking if she would advise their daughters who were about to be married. In her own practice this posed no problems. She gladly showed inexperienced girls how to stretch the hymen, explained the mode of action of the cap and chemical and introduced them to 'a new and perplexing subject—the art and science of mutually happy sexual companionship . . . The girls reappeared for check visits and reported gratefully that they *had* enjoyed their honeymoons.'[2]

In her private practice Helena was a free agent. However, she was also a paid servant of the local authority, and a different situation arose when the first patient at the North Kensington clinic asked Helena the same question. She was answerable here to the Medical Officer of Health of the Royal Borough of Kensington, through Mrs Spring Rice, and he was known to be strongly opposed to giving contraceptive advice to single women. Helena and Margery Spring Rice with five or six delegates from the clinic went to call on him, to be greeted with 'astonishment, horror and anger'.[2] In Helena's own words:

> MOH   You want me to sanction teaching contraception to unmarried girls? *Never!*
> HELENA   May I ask if you have daughters?
> MOH   I have.

[1] Personal communication to the author—20.10.80
[2] *Family Planning* (1972), 21.3.

HELENA If one of your daughters were to become engaged to be married, would you want her to have a happy marriage and choose her pregnancies when she wanted to have them?

MOH Of course!

HELENA Then she must look ahead and be prepared. Danger begins with the first intercourse.

There was a weighty silence, followed by this reply, the MOH no longer angry.

MOH Yes, of course you are right. Girls must be taught *before* they are in danger.

Thereafter the MOH was friendly and active, authorised patients to attend the clinic and saw that a regular per capita fee was paid. Prospective brides were seen from then onwards at the North Kensington clinic, and this undoubtedly influenced the FPA where opinion was still sharply divided and the question of whether or not to give contraceptive advice to unmarried girls remained a source of controversy. Helena, Joan Malleson and Dr Cecile Boyson strongly approved of doing so, but Margaret Pyke, as Chairman, whose son David has said that she would have supported the idea, had to move cautiously on a subject which engendered so much emotion as to be regarded as dynamite in the Fifties. In 1952, however, the FPA agreed at its Annual General Meeting, on the recommendation of the Medical Sub-Committee, to give advice to girls who were engaged to be married. This caused endless difficulties; some clinics wanted proof of the proposed marriage date, certificates from vicars or doctors to weed out the impostors. Official policy was to accept girls within four to eight weeks of the wedding. It was a compromise within the bounds of respectability. People like Helena continued to press for the removal of all restrictions.

As Helena put it, 'The underlying idea, never openly acknowledged, that the pleasure of sex had to be paid for by some kind of penalty was the principal, if unconscious, motive of a large number of people who opposed the new proposition.'[3] Agreement to teach unmarried women as a general principle required alteration of the constitution of the FPA. Before it could be changed a majority vote was required at the Annual General Meeting, and Lord Brain, then President, had warned the National Executive that if the vote were

[3] *Family Planning* (1972), 21. p.66.

carried it would split the FPA down the middle. A motion was drafted to which an amendment was finally passed with a satisfactory majority on 3 June 1964.

> .... That when information on contraceptive techniques is sought by the unmarried, the latter should be referred to the youth advisory centres, the setting up of which the FPA should encourage, and at which medical advice on sex problems including advice on birth control will be available.[4]

This compromise proved extremely successful. Helen Brook, who had been running the Whitfield Street clinic for Marie Stopes's legatees, included one evening session a week for unmarried girls, and in 1963 had opened the first Brook Advisory Centre for young people in adjoining premises. It was not, however, official FPA policy to give single girls advice unrestrictedly until the Family Planning Act of 1967 extended the local health authorities' powers from medical to social criteria, independent of marital status.

Helena's method of teaching prospective brides in her Weymouth Street consulting room was to give each a copy of *The Sex Factor in Marriage* and tell them to come back when they had read it. Although she had been clear in her own mind that everything they needed to know was in the book, Helena discovered that many of the girls who came had not followed the gist. 'I had not realised that however clear the printed word, it can only enter the prepared mind.' On her second visit she would make the girl read a paragraph of her book aloud while she listened, only to hear numerous girls say, 'I never saw it that way.' She then settled down to write *More About the Sex Factor in Marriage* (1947) which was originally called *Sex Fulfilment in Married Women*. She expanded and clarified those aspects which she found she had not covered adequately in her first book, in particular the role of the vagina in sexual sensitivity, claiming that this, usually absent at the beginning of sexual experience and variable in capacity, can be achieved eventually. The clitoris, she told her readers, should lead the way and say to the vagina, 'Wake up and do as we do!' Still nothing about contraception was included.

In 1968 the American science writer Edward Brecher, collecting material for his book *The Sex Researchers* (1969), came to England. He had previously written with his late wife the successful *An Analysis of*

---

[4] A. Leathard, *The Fight for Family Planning*, Macmillan, 1980

Human Sexual Response (1967) in which he had interpreted for laymen the work described by Masters and Johnson in *Human Sexual Response* (1966). In 1948 Kinsey had published *Sexual Behaviour in the Human Male*, which he followed in 1953 with *Sexual Behaviour in the Human Female*. These books were based on personal interviews with over 12,000 Americans. Kinsey's studies became the standard statistical guide to Western sexual behaviour. He and his colleagues at Indiana University also took evidence from gynaecologists who tested the sensitivity of the female genital organs to touch, as well as the reported eye-witness accounts of male and female orgasms during homosexual and heterosexual intercourse, and during masturbation.

Masters and Johnson carried the investigations into the laboratory where with the help of nearly 700 volunteers, of whom 276 were married couples, over 10,000 orgasms during intercourse or masturbation were observed. The results of this research formed the basis of *Human Sexual Response* and paved the way for the treatment programme which Masters and Johnson launched in 1959. They aimed to help men and women who were sexually inadequate—men who ejaculated prematurely, could not produce or maintain an erection; women who failed to reach orgasm and so obtain relief of tension; and all the combinations and permutations of sexual discord which the sexologists believed arose in around one in five couples.

Masters and Johnson rocked the sexual complacency of their generation and their book, *Sexual Inadequacy* (1970), became the guide for practitioners of sex therapy. Unlike Helena they disputed Freud's assertion that there were two types of female orgasm, clitoral and vaginal, and by demonstrating that there was only one type, clitoral, theoretically eliminated the guilt feelings of women who could not experience a vaginal orgasm. According to Masters and Johnson couples no longer needed to delve into the past to unlearn their bad habits.

Unlike Kinsey, and Masters and Johnson, Helena was not a research worker in the scientific sense. She knew about their writing but admitted to me to being uninterested in any therapy other than her own. The concept of sex in the laboratory was entirely foreign to her—almost inhuman. What she learnt she taught herself by her own sexual experience and that of her patients. Where she was decades ahead of her time was in asking women who consulted her for their gynaecological problems how they got on in bed with their partners, something no journalist would have mentioned in those days.

According to some reports Helena's questions were not always welcome but, having discovered the nature of the problem, she set out to educate and inform each woman according to the needs as she saw them of the individual.

The ignorance, guilt and inhibitions surrounding the unmentionable that she met and sought to dispel in her practice were infinitely greater than in the days of Kinsey or Masters and Johnson. Edward Brecher labelled her 'that pioneer of common sense in England'. He came to talk to her on his arrival in 1968 about the subject—sex—in which he had been concerned for over twenty-five years. He found her, as had many before and even more since,

> Forthright, opinionated, dominating, as well as agreeable and gracious. She was enormously sure of herself and of the rightness of her views—and she had an almost hypnotic ability to transmit this feeling of certainty to others. She didn't argue or persuade or cite evidence; she simply told me what was what. Even on points where I disagreed with her I was amazed to find myself changing my mind.[5]

Anyone who has known Helena Wright will recognise the accuracy of this thumb-nail sketch. She never appeared to doubt that her way was the best, if not the only, way, and having made up her mind she would manipulate people and situations so that things usually turned out as she wished. As Edward Brecher concluded, 'It is this remarkable power—not persuasiveness, but contagiousness of opinion—which may explain Dr Wright's ability to alter even the deepest-rooted prejudices of her patients.'

It was of course these prejudices which contributed to sexual failure, particularly the taboo which still surrounded masturbation. In *The Sex Factor in Marriage* she had written that masturbation could be 'no more than a substitute for the greater intimacy of psychological and physical intercourse between two people'. Its danger, she averred, lay not in any physical consequences but in the guilt feelings of most masturbators and the effect on later sex development. She was addressing a generation of women who had grown up to think masturbation could cause blindness, insanity and worse, and whose parents had tied their hands lest as babies they indulged in genital

[5] E. Brecher, *The Sex Researchers*, André Deutsch, 1970.

play. She could well have cited the view, sometimes expressed today, that '95 per cent do and 5 per cent won't say'.

It was by using a form of masturbation that, as much as ten years before Masters and Johnson began adapting their laboratory findings to therapeutic uses, Helena had developed a simple procedure which she described in *More About the Sex Factor in Marriage* (1947):

> By laying her hand on the man's hand the woman rhythmically guides his hand over the parts of the vulva in ways she finds erotically arousing. In doing this she teaches him her preferred clitoral rhythm while learning herself. It is not necessary for her to think or plan; her clitoris and the sensitive area around it respond instantly to touch; all she has to do is to move her husband's fingers instinctively and freely, and to go on with the movements for as long as she feels pleasurable sensations.

This had impressed Edward Brecher, who noted that Helena's teaching was particularly applicable for women whose aversion to masturbation was warping their whole sexual outlook.

> Dr Wright's approach . . . is aimed with exquisite precision at their problems . . . The impact of this procedure on psychological attitudes is clear. The woman whose responses are inhibited by fear of 'losing control' can relax in the knowledge that *she* remains in control. The woman whose sexual hang-up is an infantile need to have something magical done *to* her and *for* her, finds herself in a position where she herself *must* take the lead. The man's attitudes, too, are affected in significant ways. Thus what appears at first blush to be a gimmick is in fact a procedure for the effective re-structuring of a couple's attitudes.[6]

Edward Brecher's comments highlight Helena's own personality, her attitude to sex and her instinctive need and ability to dominate a situation, in this case the sex relationship. Only the naive would not perceive that Helena evolved the technique described by trial and error in response to personal frustration, and was passing on her findings to others in need of help. As she was to write twenty years later:

[6] Brecher, *op.cit.*

It is to be hoped that long familiarity with the new ideas will save all but the unalterably orthodox from risking marriage between virgins . . . a marriage between two virgins is asking for the maximum risk of sexual disharmony.[7]

Throughout her life Helena considered herself primarily an educationalist and increasingly she wanted to change the opinions of the public, the churches and the law. Fundamentally she regarded it as her duty to teach women to space their families but she also wanted to teach medical students. She had an opportunity when in April 1962 she was the guest writer in the *Middlesex Hospital Journal* on family planning and chose to raise among other subjects that of sexual activity among unmarried students:

That sympathy and respect should be given to the sexual energies of the unmarried is a comparatively new idea, and still inevitably shocking and disturbing to the conventionally minded. We who are trying to alter the old ideas for new and better ones must not be lacking in respect and understanding of the basis of the sexual conventions as are generally held. Before the invention of reliable contraception those conventions were necessary for the stability of family life. But now with the advent of contraception better prospects are slowly becoming available. The object of teaching contraceptive technique to young couples who are seriously thinking of marriage, is to give them a chance to find out in private and dignified circumstances (which should ideally be provided by the parents of the two) whether or not they are good sexual companions, and so to increase as much as possible their chances of staying happily together for life.

Without going into the rights and wrongs of freedom for sexual intercourse among students not intending to marry, the article concluded that:

It is the inescapable duty that some relevant authority should undertake to supply detailed and reliable information about conception and contraception to everyone in its charge who might become in danger of either causing or receiving an unwanted pregnancy.

---

[7] Helena Wright, *Sex and Society: A New Code of Sexual Behaviour*, 1968.

This was altogether too much for the *Church Times*. An editorial called on the Governors of the Middlesex Hospital to issue a public disclaimer and to 'ensure that nothing of the kind is allowed to occur again'. The hospital secretary rightly replied that as the journal was run and edited by students and young doctors, the Board of Governors had no jurisdiction in the matter.

Helena was, of course, quite unrepentant. She told a *Daily Express* reporter that she knew the article would cause some controversy, but that she regarded discussion of such matters as 'very healthy'. Peter Wright is said to have sighed when told of the *Church Times*'s protest. He told the *Express* reporter that 'perhaps the article was written a little too provocatively and was a little unwise', but added loyally that he agreed with his wife's views, saying truthfully that she had 'very many years of experience with these problems'.

Helena's final book, *Sex and Society: A New Code of Sexual Behaviour* (1968), took four years to write and was the least successful from the publisher's point of view. It sold less than 4,000 copies and went out of print in 1974. It was the only book for which she had difficulty in finding a publisher; the editorial staff of George Allen and Unwin who finally took it were not unanimous about accepting a book which advocated extramarital sexual activity. As she wrote:

> Perhaps the most difficult and controversial suggestion contained in the new code is the one which proposes that extramarital sexual friendships entered into by both husbands and wives need not upset or damage the married relationship in any way, but rather could enrich both partners and add depth to the marriage.

Moreover she considered it unreasonable

> . . . to expect two individuals to promise in a religious ceremony to undertake with one another and with no one else for the rest of their lives something of which neither has had any experience . . . In no other undertaking would it occur to anyone to make such a blind promise . . . Until the advent of contraception there could have been no other course of action. Thus the strictness of the demand appears to be justified by the importance of the issues at stake.

Helena believed that 'life-long restriction of sexual activity with one individual is not only unnatural, but impossible to maintain'. She did, however, elaborate a code for maintaining the responsibility and status of marriage.

(1) No new sex relationship should cause damage or distress to an existing one.

(2) No financial advantage to either side should accrue in any sex relationship which is outside marriage.

(3) Financially dependent individuals must not enter into a sex relationship of which their source of support would disapprove, with the possible exception of marriage.

(4) Fidelity to one partner to the exclusion of all other sex relationships must not be demanded.

(5) Neither possessiveness nor jealousy must enter into a sex relationship.

(6) Marriage and parenthood should be the only sex relationships which are public property. All other kinds should be of concern only to the individuals involved.

Helena was only preaching what she had practised for years. Her first cousin, Gunther Lowenfeld, who admired her and had every reason to be grateful to her for housing and helping him financially as a refugee from Nazi Germany in 1938, has described her as 'clear-minded and natural' but he thought she had 'the most extraordinary outlook on sex, marriage and life . . . She must have had numerous men friends . . . whom she thought were sexually blocked and it was her duty to show them how to change, and to teach them to live nicely sexually. She always said her husband was a dear, but they seldom spent a weekend together. Helena went always to the country house of a good friend.'

One of Helena's early extramarital relationships involved a young married doctor who had been one of Peter's students in China, and who greatly admired him. He used to visit the Wrights regularly after their return in 1927 to England. From letters written to Helena from China after his first trip in 1928, it is clear that she had contributed to his sexual education during his time in London.

Back home, he had written to Helena that his sexual life in China was not very satisfactory because 'the art was not right' and he had failed many times in spite of his excitement. 'What I need most is the respond.' But on 1 July 1929 L F reported progress; intercourse had improved. Using the sex methods Helena had taught him he now found family life more satisfactory, 'I have never enjoyed the sexual life so much as now.' But it had not 'reached the high point, as the opposite side is too conservative . . . I do not believe there will be anyone else besides you who will do such noble and gentle love to me. How much I appreciate your gentle and thoughtful deed which you did to me when I was in England.'

On 15 March 1930, L F wrote:

> The time we had in England is so vivid to me. I can remember every detail. The time we had in Edinburgh is so sweet to me. O the sensation of touch, the sensation of your respond, the light, the atmosphere and everything were so harmonious which made me happy that I can never forget in all my life. I am always thankful to you as you have rendered me such an opportunity to enjoy the beauty of love and the art to carry it out . . . You are my ideal woman both physically and spiritually. But I cannot expect any more from you besides intimate friendship. I am thankful there is a woman in the world whom I love and trust, and to whom I can tell everything about myself. I am always proud of our relationship as you have never cheat[ed] your husband and I never my friend [Peter]. This is the thing that I have great respect to you and a comfort to myself. My thoughts have always been with you. I love you more and more still.
>
> Your L F

It was perhaps ironic that the one sexual aspect on which Helena the surrogate failed to enlighten her pupil was birth control. L F referred to this in 1930 as 'an absolute failure'; six children were already too many and L F asked Helena to send his wife some pills.

Modern sex therapists would not accept that Helena was a therapeutic surrogate. Her services were rendered on her own generous terms rather than those which Masters and Johnson first introduced as one aspect of their therapy; this has never been used as extensively in Britain as in the United States where it is now gaining momentum and acceptance, while being still regarded in Britain with the greatest reserve. The American sex surrogate is a trained, professional woman who is paid to treat men, although a minority of women have been treated recently by male practitioners with all the inherent potential complications. Helena's contribution was part of her general sexual philosophy which was to apply throughout her life to her relationships with her friends.

American sexologists use the word 'surrogate' to distinguish therapists in that branch from prostitutes. Not so Helena: the ethical considerations which have concerned American sex practitioners for over twenty-five years would not have been covered by the code she postulated in *Sex and Society*. Moreover she would not qualify today as an acceptable surrogate, whose services must never be contaminated by feelings of emotion, least of all affection. What she did satisfy was her own code.

Today when stable and not-so-stable relationships are common among the young, Helena's views will not seem particularly extraordinary. But when she first practised in England the country was still adjusting to the devastating effect Marie Stopes's revolutionary ideas had produced. *Lady Chatterley's Lover* was banned in England in 1928 and Lawrence's paintings confiscated in 1929. It is a tribute to Helena that she was able to achieve so much that was contrary to conventional opinion of the day. Some of her own 'respectability' must have been due to her medical position in the world, but by the time she wrote *Sex and Society*, Helena, then nearly eighty, was blatantly out to shock as well as to help. She knew her views were unacceptable to many people. For years she had told her patients they should maintain their marriages rather than break up the family, but if sexual compatibility had been lost, it was better to seek sexual happiness elsewhere —though not on the doorstep.

Dr Jean Infield, who worked with her for many years, said Helena regarded a lover as a form of therapy. 'She did not tell women to go out and look for another man, but her views brought them up in their tracks.' According to Dr Infield, the women would say, 'Oh, I couldn't do that; I love my husband too much,' but they would take a new look at themselves and realise that Helena was, as it were, legitimising extramarital solace. It was as if she were saying, 'If you are so miserably unhappy sexually with your husband, have the sex somewhere else but be happy with your husband in other ways.'

Of course, Helena's philosophy elicited complaints from various directions in relation to the views expressed in *Sex and Society*. A 'most deeply grateful ex-patient' wrote, 30 March 1970, that *Sex and Society* made her 'infinitely sad'. She could probably argue with something on every page; had Helena realised what her code would do for women?

In removing the protection of virtue it removes the choice with it . . . Are you quite determined to take away the beautiful, glorious magic of an unique experience with one person loved beyond others? There is no doubt that if it ceases to be ideal this permanent relationship will cease to exist . . . I am just wondering if a close look at your own ideals might not lead to the discovery that you have allowed safe contraception to become your god? I offer these observations in affection and hope they will be so received.

Helena had indeed made contraception her 'god' and some might say that this act of uncritical faith may not have been justified. There are feminists in society today who assert that contraception gives men unreasonable access to women's bodies by making a woman feel churlish if she refuses intercourse. A journalist who put this point to Helena in the last year of her life got short shrift. Helena could not accept that contraception might be a two-edged tool, because it was an essential part of her character to remain in control whenever possible of any situation. The same would go for Marie Stopes who considered a man who forced his wife to have intercourse unwillingly was guilty of rape, a view which has been canvassed some fifty years later by the feminists who followed Marie. Helena's philosophy, expressed typically to another interviewer on her ninetieth birthday was, 'You like music, but you don't always want to listen to Mozart.' When inviting the reporter to visit her in the country, Helena told her to bring her lover 'regardless of the fact,' as the girl said, 'that I might not have one'.

If she had doubts Helena never expressed them to me. She assumed, characteristically, that just as she had maintained happy and loving relationships while keeping her marriage intact, others could do the same. Only someone devoid of the baser emotions of envy and jealousy could have achieved this goal.

[10]
Friends and Relations

Helena heaved a sigh of relief at leaving Hounslow early in 1928, and the Wrights' new family home at Randolph Crescent in Maida Vale proved a success. Her mother, who had always liked Peter, could now come and visit them unaccompanied by Frank. Return visits to Hounslow were harmonious, Frank's manners having apparently improved.

The house was—as Helena had intended—large. She had never lifted a duster in her life, let alone a broom. Apart from 'ordering the meals'—a solemn daily conference, and 'checking the accounts', a farcical weekly ceremony, she left all the domestic arrangements of the new ménage to the cook. The French nurse, Mademoiselle Mullié, ran the nurseries at the top of the house and acted as self-appointed watch-dog on the kitchen staff. Helena simply had to keep them all happy and see that Peter was properly looked after. As her son Michael said at her memorial gathering, she gave her husband

> . . . truly loving affection and respect but kept strictly in balance with her other strong relationships and professional activities. This was shown at home by her concern for his comfort and his preferences—the family breakfast and dinner were organised precisely for his convenience—by her obvious affection and real interest in all his doings when she was with him, by the endless patience and precision with which she would darn an enormous hole in one of his socks . . . She offered him throughout their life together the same freedom to develop separate interests and separate strong personal relationships that she included in her own immensely full and varied life. But looking back over those years it seems to me that he could never achieve the same detachment and balance between the separate parts of his life that she could in hers; that, extraordinary experience though it must have been to be married to Helena, he

175

would in the upshot have been happier with a more single-minded and conventional wife.[1]

Almost as soon as they had moved to their new home Helena's practice began to grow, as did her public commitments. She was soon fully embarked on the course she was to follow henceforth. This meant that she was increasingly at the mercy of her domestic staff, usually loyal and generous women. There were, of course, exceptions. In China her servants had cheated her in small ways, even on one occasion renting out their sleeping accommodation, and regularly taking a rake-off on the food bills. A similar pattern developed at Randolph Crescent. One cook invented twenty-three different ways of swindling her in a single week's accounts. Helena told me with a wry smile that she first learnt of this extortion from the French nurse who also told her that her butler was in the habit of taking one of her suitcases full of coal round to his mother every evening. For several months a Portuguese couple, working as cook and butler, kept their child in the house hidden from Helena. When this was discovered they expressed regret but explained they were saving up to buy a house in Portugal and had therefore also had to cook the books.

According to an old friend, Mary Ainslie, Helena was, however, never without servants and had them when no one else did: 'They were devoted to her, like the secretaries. She was very good at getting people to do things for her and made people work for her. She used to talk to them as equals and they loved it.' Mrs Ainslie had been the first wife of Dr Edward Griffith (always known as 'G') whom Helena had taught at Telford Road. 'She had seen he had beautiful hands and realised he was worth teaching and would not upset the patients,' recalled Mrs Ainslie. 'G admired her although he used to get annoyed with her and laugh at her, but she was much more intelligent than he was.' The families became friends and often spent their holidays together. The first time they rented a house together at Perranporth, Cornwall, Helena arrived first and by the time the Griffith family turned up, Helena had allocated all the bedrooms. Helena was bossy and intimidated Mrs Griffith, as she then was, but she came to love Helena. 'Her warmth, love and outgoing personality will never be equalled,' Mrs Ainslie has said. 'She was kind and practical and once walked miles over the moor when staying with a friend on Exmoor, to see if she could help a woman who was ill in a farmhouse.'

[1] Michael Wright at the Friends Meeting House, 25.5.82

Mrs Ainslie has described Helena in those days as having 'very bright eyes, she always wore pince-nez glasses, which she kept taking on and off, which was rather unnerving. She was not pretty at all, but was striking-looking rather than good-looking. She had a beautiful aquiline nose and a mobile mouth; she was stocky but not fat, and was always trying to keep her weight down. She was not keen on clothes, although she could be tidy.' According to Mrs Ainslie, Helena was quite uninhibited and would walk about the hotel corridors in her petticoat. Mrs Ainslie's chief impression was of Helena's powers of perception. 'She would catch on to an idea, could grasp a point at once and always knew the score. She always had a lot on and was usually in a frightful rush or else, on holiday, she would want to sleep all the afternoon.'[2]

Helena and Peter had bought 5 Randolph Crescent with a building society loan and a mortgage. Almost continuously for forty-five years the Wrights existed on an overdraft, apparently with neither apprehension nor anxiety. The only person who seems to have been worried was one of their secretaries, Olive Stewart. The secretaries worked from the house, as Helena preferred, unlike the other consultants, not to have them around in her consulting room at Weymouth Street because she thought their presence might disturb the confidentiality between herself and her patients. A porter let the patients in and Helena showed them out. Their first secretary, Marjorie Hay, organised a system whereby the files with patients' cards and notes were kept at Randolph Crescent and returned there after each day's consultation.

The secretaries also dealt with the domestic finances and paid the servants' wages, and when Olive first expressed some anxiety about her employers' overdraft, Helena typically dissociated herself from the problem and sent Olive round to see the bank manager. She came back with the information that the bank regarded the Drs Wright's business as a 'nice lively account'.

Olive need not have worried. *The Sex Factor in Marriage* soon brought in substantial royalties, including the overseas sales and translation rights. When the first cheque for the American royalties arrived, Helena had to ask Marjorie Hay to tell her if she was seeing aright—it was for £1,065 and she could not believe her eyes. The American publishers had raised doubts that the book might contravene the Comstock Law. Helena might have lost her £1,065 had she

[2] Personal communication to the author—7.4.82.

not written herself to the objector, telling him that if he would 'sit down all alone and read the manuscript from cover to cover' he would find 'no reference to birth control'. A harder problem proved to be the piracy of the book in Canada when pages from the American edition were photographed and unlawfully reproduced.

In the early days Helena went to work on the Number 6 bus and it was some time before the Wrights decided to buy a secondhand car—a Morris—which in order to avoid leaving the lights on they parked in a mews and not outside their home. If Peter needed the car and Helena could not get it to him, she might leave it somewhere for him to pick up. After one occasion when it spent the night in the middle of Regent Street, awaiting collection, they decided to become a two-car family, buying one for Helena and a large Buick for Peter.

The atmosphere at home was a mixture of the conventional and the unusual. As children the boys did not know many other families since Helena had no friends among women engaged in social activities and was seldom at home, although she tried to get back for nursery tea and sometimes succeeded. According to Michael Wright he and his brothers became a rather self-sufficient unit, taking it for granted that they would be left to nannies and servants while their mother was busy with her professional life. He has described their mother's relationship with her children as:

> . . . one of detached affection and strictly egalitarian between the four of us. She was never possessive nor was she resentful of the time and energy needed when her family took its turn for her attention. Memories include journeys through a December London fog to let the four of us loose to choose our own Christmas presents in Hamleys; and the endless care with which she planned the family summer holidays—a farm in Norfolk, a whole schoolhouse in Perranporth, and later, more adventurously, a carload of teenage family and friends across the breadth of Europe; or nearer home when under her amused tolerance four scratchy children tried to agree on a film for a wet Saturday afternoon.[3]

The four boys all went to what one of them has described as 'the best of the bad schools'. Helena held what she considered to be 'advanced' ideas about education and Michael was the only one to receive an

[3] Michael Wright at the Friends Meeting House, 25.5.82

'orthodox' one. Helena made her first mistake, as she freely admitted, with their eldest son, Beric. He was ten when they moved to Randolph Crescent and he went initially to Dartington Hall, then run by two unconventional educationalists, Dorothy and Leonard Elmhirst, who believed in 'promoting the liberty of the child'. A year later the Wrights discovered that Beric's weekly programme consisted of five woodwork, two basket-making and three pottery sessions, and that he was learning nothing else of educational value. Helena's complaints went unheeded, the Elmhirsts telling her they were not prepared to ask Beric to do anything he did not wish to do. Finding Dartington then 'as rigid as Eton', as Helena put it, she took him away and sent him to school in Bembridge in the Isle of Wight.

In 1930 Helena, lunching as a guest in All Souls, Oxford, found herself sitting next to a quiet young man, Bruce McFarlane, a fellow of Magdalen who was later to play an important part in her life. Helena talked about China, and her neighbour offered to take a group of her Chinese student friends round Magdalen. From then on their friendship blossomed. Within three years Bruce as an educationalist professed himself dissatisfied with Beric's school reports and advised his parents to send him to Manchester Grammar School although the boy had flourished and been perfectly happy at Bembridge. Helena took Bruce McFarlane's advice to Beric's great annoyance, and he never did well at Manchester, leaving within a year.

After these three 'failures' Helena tried to find a co-educational school to compensate for the lack of sisters and female society, and sent Beric when he was sixteen to St Christopher's, Letchworth. In addition to being co-educational it was also vegetarian and so could be considered 'advanced'. From there he went to University College and Hospital, where he qualified in 1942. During the war he rose to the rank of major in the army as a specialist in physiology, working mainly on the design of the interior of tanks. After demobilisation he returned to University College Hospital until 1952 when he joined Shell, and following two overseas tours of duty, he became a Fellow of the Royal College of Surgeons in 1955, but abandoned surgery in favour of the Institute of Directors. There in 1958 he founded the Research Unit, which became the Institute's Medical Centre, which was taken over by BUPA in London in 1970. He finally became Chairman of the BUPA Medical Centre in London and a director of BUPA Insurance. By then he had parted from Joyce Normand, a veterinary surgeon whom he had married as a student in 1941 on the strength of his part-time job in a pregnancy diagnosis laboratory. He married Susan Bullock in 1967.

Christopher, the second boy, was subject to an even more varied education than Beric, involving six schools altogether. At ten he too went to Bembridge but was removed with Beric on Bruce's advice, sent to Dauntsey's, and then Gordonstoun at the same time that Prince Philip was at the school. He appeared to have no intellectual interests, showing ability only in physical activities including sailing and later flying. Before entering him for Gordonstoun, Helena invited the celebrated headmaster, Kurt Hahn, to meet her at Brown's Hotel in London, and warned him about her son's 'irrepressible individualism'. According to Helena Hahn smiled his 'conceited Germanic smile' and said that her son was 'just the sort of boy we like to have at Gordonstoun', but Hahn later reported that meeting Christopher was the first time he had been interviewed by a boy. After a year Helena asked Hahn how Christopher was doing, to which he replied that Christopher was not amenable to discipline and 'unschoolable'. When she asked Christopher the same question his reply shook her even more: 'I know who his spies are, so lying is no good,' he told his mother.

This was enough for Helena to shift him once again, this time to Millfield. Here the headmaster, Mr Myers, miraculously came up with a solution. Her sister, Margaret Lowenfeld, had already told Helena she should put the unhappy boy on a farm. Myers, at Millfield, gave Christopher a horse and told him he was to be entirely responsible for grooming and feeding it. It was his salvation. In spite of hunting two or three times a week the boy got the equivalent of two O levels before leaving the school.

Christopher wanted to join the Fleet Air Arm at the outbreak of war but there were no vacancies, so he tried Fighter Command and was accepted. In contrast to his school career he did well there and got high marks in his training examinations without, according to his brother Michael, doing a stroke of work. He would spend one or two nights a week in London night clubs, sometimes driving up in one car and back in another, having swapped cars with someone else during the evening. At the end of his training he got his 'wings', but not, to his chagrin, a commission. Perhaps the fact that on one occasion he had landed a Tiger Moth in the middle of Nottingham race track had influenced his masters. When Christopher heard he had not been commissioned, he disappeared for some months.

Shortly before the war Peter had bought a fifty-foot cabin cruiser, the *Cairngorm*, which slept six, and much of the family's energies had gone into fitting her out. It was Peter's pride and joy, and he used it at weekends and for family holidays in which Helena sometimes joined. He kept the *Cairngorm* on the Thames and in 1940 after the fall of Dunkirk, when all the little boats were mobilised for the evacuation, he set off eagerly in the flotilla with Dr Edward Griffith, then an Aldershot general practitioner. They reached Ramsgate only to learn that Peter's duties lay at his hospital. To his great sorrow a crew from the Royal Thames Yacht Club with an elated Edward Griffith took the boat across the Channel, while Peter made his own disconsolate way back to London from Ramsgate.

The *Cairngorm* brought sixty men back from the Normandy beaches. Peter and Helena with Marjorie Hay and Freda Bromhead joined the cheering crowds which welcomed the return procession of little boats up the Thames. The *Cairngorm* was in poor shape after her arduous trips when the Navy handed her back at Charing Cross Pier some days later. Peter immediately took her up to Chertsey for a refit, but more disappointment followed. The Navy had liked the boat so much that they commandeered her for the rest of the war.

About three months later Christopher surfaced. He rang his father up with the surprising news that he was now in the Navy as a leading seaman. 'Strange coincidence,' he said, 'I'm on your boat', though how he had achieved this feat was never vouchsafed. He resumed his night life as described by Michael Wright, then up at Oxford, who joined Christopher in a number of his exploits:

> He would now appear for the evening in a stunning tailor-made AB uniform sporting RAF wings, normally worn only by an RAF officer, enough to intrigue any girl. The rest of his war would read like an Evelyn Waugh novel, a snakes and ladders of promotions, postings and courses involving everything but active service. At an Officers' Training Course he got up a successful hockey team to play the neighbouring station, but was later seen dancing with the Station Commander's wife, so back to the ranks.
>
> Personal communication to the author—8.5.83

He was then given the job of Admiral's Boatman at Portsmouth, and attached to a transit camp to ferry senior naval officers between their ships and the shore. After eighteen months he applied to join a radar mechanics' course and was posted to an aircraft carrier in the Indian Ocean. He finished up as a petty officer in charge of the disposal of naval property in Trincomalee, where he relieved his boredom by playing a guitar on deck.

Bruce McFarlane had been responsible for recommending the Dragon School at Oxford for Michael, whom Helena believed was the most intelligent of her sons. He got a scholarship to the Dragon and then one to Sedbergh. From there he went up to Magdalen as an Exhibitioner, to read physics for two years on a government scheme intended to promote radar design and development, and came out with a BA in physics in 1943. At the TRE (Telecommunications Research Establishment) at Malvern he became concerned with the problems, amongst others, of aircraft landing in bad weather. He was later to qualify in medicine at Oxford in 1954, became a Fellow of the Royal College of Surgeons of Edinburgh in 1964, and a consultant surgeon.

For Michael school life was comparatively uncomplicated, but this was not so in the case of the fourth boy, Adrian. His physical disability made things difficult for him and for his parents and it says as much for them as for Adrian himself that he emerged with no evident resentment for the raw deal life had dealt him. He managed to go through conventional schooling, first at a pre-preparatory school in Orme Square in London, then at a preparatory school in Malvern, before going on to St Christopher's, Letchworth. At St Christopher's his friends taught him to bicycle and he was able to ride all over London on his own, a feat which few spastics are even allowed to attempt. At Magdalen College he was a pupil of Bruce McFarlane and took an Oxford honours degree in history. Because he could not write clearly he was given extra time in which to type his examination papers, supervised by a don in a side room. Adrian eventually went on to the London School of Economics to undertake historical research under H. L. Beales, ending up in a successful solicitor's practice.

Adrian was greatly helped by Miss Margaret Kirschner, a physical re-educationalist to whom he went for treatment two or three times a week in the holidays over several years. Miss Kirschner taught Adrian from the age of twelve consciously to control and co-ordinate his movements. He has said, and Helena confirmed this, that she was the only person who was able to help him at all, and Adrian has remained grateful to her all his life. She had first met him 1933 when she arrived in England as a refugee from Nazi Germany. She had known the Adolf

Lowenfelds ever since, as a child of four, she had stayed at Chrzanow with her family, her father, an ear, nose and throat surgeon, being a life-long friend of Adolf's. The English Lowenfelds were not at Chrzanow that summer. Thirty years later Adolf's daughter Rösel gave her an introduction to her London cousins when she was leaving Germany, warning Margaret (known in Germany as Grete) Kirschner, 'If you are in with one you will be out with the other.' And so it proved. Both Helena and Margaret helped her to get established in England but with Margaret Lowenfeld she developed a close and lasting co-operation.

Miss Kirschner soon realised the accuracy of Rösel's assessment of the relationship of the two sisters. They were never close and often at loggerheads. Their only common interest appeared to be extra-sensory perception (ESP) on which they would talk for hours. Outwardly shyer than Helena, who inhibited her, Margaret could be as autocratic and dogmatic as her sister. She was apt to be moody, emotional and often depressed. She envied her sister's worldly success and resented the fact that she herself was always short of money. She was entirely dependent on her small private practice which disappeared when Margaret wanted to take time off to write or study, to visit Jung in Zurich or Margaret Mead in America.

Each of the sisters had inherited £30,000 on their mother's death, under the Quicke trust, but Margaret was not financially adept and was given to borrowing sums of money from Helena. Her achievements, though different, were at least as considerable as Helena's, and she had received even greater recognition in the United States than in Britain through Margaret Mead, who described Margaret Lowenfeld as 'one of the great pioneers'. As their father once said, 'Madge has the brains and originality but Helena the capability.' Margaret was an innovator, Helena an ingenious adapter of the original ideas of others. Towards the end of her life, Helena came to accept that Margaret had been 'a celebrity', but once told me that she and her sister were actually, like their father, 'genetic freaks'.

Helena had greeted Margaret Kirschner with the words 'You're German so you talk about sex,' and sent her to treat one of her patients in Cambridge who had marital problems about which, apart from the language barrier, Miss Kirschner was almost totally ignorant, and the only thing she and her patient had in common was that both could play the flute. Helena then found Miss Kirschner a holiday job with two children near where the Wrights were staying at Mudeford, where she first met Adrian, a silent little boy with his nanny. Back in London, she gradually built up a practice and also worked for thirty years as a therapist with Margaret Lowenfeld at the Institute of Child Psychology. There she taught disturbed children to be aware of physical happenings and to discover their own physical potential, thus enabling them to combat their physical shortcomings such as asthma or spinal deformity, and to use their bodies freely as a natural means of self-expression. In this way, physical activity became an accessory in the understanding and treatment of children's emotional problems. Among the doctors she worked for in London she met Joan Malleson whose tense patients she taught to relax.

Helena, who had seen how successful Miss Kirschner was proving with Adrian, employed her at Telford Road, primarily to treat women with prolapse after childbirth. At the clinic Miss Kirschner developed her own method of showing these women how to re-educate the lax muscles of the pelvic floor, and how to build up a correct posture. When I met her she was over eighty and the flexibility of her own joints amazed me.

Miss Kirschner confirmed my own impression that Helena was not able to accept the full implication of Adrian's disability. She had told Miss Kirschner, as she had told me, that his birth was an easy delivery—just one or two pains—contrary to the evidence she had provided in her letter to her mother, where it is clear that it had been a medically induced and a medically maintained long confinement for a fourth baby. Helena disagreed with Peter's diagnosis that Adrian had a consequent spastic diplegia and used merely to say that as a child he was 'rather backward and had difficulty with his movements', an example of genuine self-deception and evidence of how Helena could blind herself psychologically to a situation she could not deal with; for her it then ceased to exist.

Adrian overcame his difficulties by his own insight and perseverance. He had an acute sense of humour which must have helped. One day at a bus stop a woman came up to him and pressed a shilling into his spastic hand: 'Buy yourself something nice,' she said. 'Do I really look as if my parents don't earn a large income?' he asked Miss Kirschner endearingly.

At home, in spite of her unorthodox views, Helena demanded a degree of outwardly conventional behaviour and her children grew up in an adult Edwardian environment. Strict punctuality at meals was demanded. Sharing their beds with their girl-friends when they were

older was acceptable, even encouraged, but holding hands in public
was frowned upon. The house in Randolph Crescent reminded Miss
Freda Bromhead, who adopted the Wrights as her war work and
became their housekeeper and a permanent family friend, of house-
holds that might have featured in the novels of Margaret Drabble or
Elizabeth Jane Howard. Freda Bromhead was a writer herself, and
before the war had run a small picture gallery. At Randolph Crescent
she found:

> . . . a spaciousness about the house . . . an impression of
> warmth (although in fact it was rather a cold house) and
> liberality. Parquet floors, high ceilings . . . the entrance hall a
> big room in itself; Chippendale chairs, a silk Persian rug on the
> wall . . . bibelots on a round table in the window (all having to
> be lifted and dusted . . .) a metal belt set with turquoise and
> pearl—Eastern or Turkish? Other ornaments of marble or
> ivory.
> Silver birds on the large oval pie-crust-edged dining table with
> flowers in the middle and a silver dog, valuable silver candle-
> sticks on the sideboard below the great Victorian landscape by
> Leader. Could it have been five foot by four foot? Blue Persian
> tiles. Chinese cabinets with embroideries and silks in them.
> All sorts of people were welcomed and accepted. In the war a
> bomber pilot on leave after bombing Berlin sat at table next to a
> conscientious objector—equal tolerance on both sides. Chinese,
> German, Czechoslovak, French, Polish, Indian and Belgian
> visitors, an Oxford don, a music student, a Viennese doctor.
> Helena once brought a Czechoslovakian soldier, Evgen, home
> after midnight. Returning from visiting Bruce McFarlane at
> Oxford, she had heard the boy asking the ticket collector at
> Paddington where he could get a bed for the night. 'Come along
> with me,' she had said.
> The young men who came to stay were sometimes arrogant,
> leaving messages for their friends with the secretaries. People
> were welcomed generously but not uncritically. The young men
> who didn't write bread-and-butter letters were not invited
> again. (They thought that as it was such an unconventional
> household, there was no need for the formal courtesies.) They
> also had to accept some surprises such as Helena sitting down by
> one at breakfast and saying, 'Now you look intelligent. How

would you like to be a sperm donor? This is what it would
entail . . . '

Personal communication to the author—14.1.80

Freda often found it hard to catch Helena in order to discuss the
household arrangements; the interview might take place while Helena
was in her bath in the morning, before she left for her first appointment at Weymouth Street. Helena was always up early and Miss
Bromhead remembered her in a silk dressing-gown, mixing muesli at
a side table. Muesli had recently been introduced into England from
the Swiss Bircher Benner Clinic by her cousin by marriage Claire
Lowenfeld who about this time was also promoting rose-hip syrup.
Helena, cheerfully voluble, would take her place at the end of the table
while Peter sat at the other end 'always at low ebb, needing coffee,
honey—and silence'.

On Wednesday evenings Helena would come home exhausted after
her North Kensington clinic. These nights were inviolate, when she
would not want to talk or telephone. Invariably on Wednesday she
had her supper on a tray, sherry, baked custard made with her weekly
rationed egg, and fruit. At other times Helena was extremely active.
In the evenings there might be table-turning sessions with the ouija
board. Helena believed increasingly in the paranormal and had
inherited an interest in spiritualism from her mother. Before Alice
died in September 1930, she and Helena had agreed that whoever
'passed over' first would communicate with the other. Helena was
convinced she had received the message of Alice's death before the
news was confirmed by the nurse who was caring for her in her last
illness. Others believe that Helena had once again deceived herself.
She may also have deceived others, and one frequent participant in
the letter and glass-moving sessions has testified that he had seen
Helena give the glass a surreptitious shove. Her customary manipula-
tion of her pendulum never convinced me, although she herself
fervently believed in its diagnostic powers, even accepting its advice as
to whether or not her plants needed water. Peter, according to Freda
Bromhead, never took part in the table-turning sessions, saying he
was 'an agnostic' in this respect.

Christmas was spent in the Lowenfeld tradition—the great Christmas tree was decorated on Christmas Eve, followed by a Polish dinner
of lobster bisque, carp and white pudding with poppy seeds. Conventional English Christmas dinner was eaten the next day, served on the

lace cloth Helena kept for special occasions. She took endless trouble over choosing and doing up her Christmas gifts but never sent cards, although she herself received hundreds.

From Freda Bromhead I got my first intimate picture of the shadowy figure who was married to this extraordinary woman, and to whom Helena always referred during our many conversations in affectionate terms as 'kind', 'good', 'clever' or 'wise'. Freda Bromhead found Peter 'charming with children except his own, from whom he was rather detached'. Neither of the Wrights was in her opinion a particularly good parent, although extremely good, by contrast, with children other than their own. At least one of the Wright boys resented Helena's absence from their school functions, and the fact that she never came down to see him at half-term like other parents.

Freda Bromhead had met the Wrights through her friend Marjorie Hay, their first secretary, the daughter of a celebrated cardiologist in Liverpool, and the sister of John Hay, the distinguished professor of paediatrics. The first time Freda went to Randolph Crescent Peter Wright took her down to the basement to see a cat and her kittens. She appreciated his many kindnesses during her stay in their household. He was interested in the arts, especially the ballet, a world in which he had many friends. The Wrights, after dining at home, often took Freda and Marjorie Hay to concerts, for which they might have bought blocks of eight to twelve seats. Peter gave Freda a season ticket to the Proms; on Christmas morning he would take her and some of her friends to swim at the Lansdowne Club, and on Sundays they might go skating at Queen's ice rink. Freda thought Peter was kinder to his non-paying patients than to his richer ones, and she remembered him walking up and down the big drawing-room, communing with himself and muttering, 'But my relation to society is not that of a surgeon.' 'What is it then?' she asked, but he did not reply. He was to have many doubts about the prospects for the National Health Service when it was first introduced, and feared it would undermine the relationship between doctor and patient.

Marjorie Hay left the Wrights to marry a man much older than herself who had been married before, Arnold Silcock. It turned out disastrously, but she was still in love with Silcock when she left him. She went back to the Wrights for comfort, and Helena took her on as a temporary assistant to Olive Stewart, to type her books and her letters to patients. Helena introduced Marjorie Hay to a new world where, as she has said:

Sex was discussed like mutton recipes and with as much gla-
mour—salutary for me, the miserable romantic. Peter was
rarely around and dictated very little. If he did sit down in the
study he would be reading—philosophy, history, poetry. He
said little but lent me books, and occasionally he would take me
to a concert or the Russian ballet—a whole new exciting world
for me because I had never been able to afford seats for either
and knew nothing of the world of free London music . . . The
impact of Baronova, Rhiabushinka, Massine and the others was
indescribable, and the fact that when Massine hurt his leg in, I
think, *The Three-Cornered Hat*, Peter went backstage to help,
made me more fully aware of Peter as a surgeon, in touch with
worlds into which most medical people never enter.

From the ballet or the concert we would drift into a Soho
restaurant. There I learnt to appreciate good food, good drink
and above all Peter's immediate rapport with all kinds of people.
He would tell me of China—how he once stopped a dangerous
riot by making people laugh . . . We would sometimes go on
from Soho, however late, to the French or German hospitals to
see a patient on whom he had operated that morning. On the
way home he would talk about the patients and the nursing
nuns . . . Each patient was a person, a whole person, not a collection of symptoms—a continuation for me of my father's
ethics.

Personal communication to the author—29.4.81

Olive had found Marjorie a flat in the same block as her own in St
John's Wood and Peter, who was much less busy than Helena, helped
her to furnish it with materials from Heals and Libertys, which he
would pay for if she could not. As Marjorie described it:

The new flat, very gradually, became a 'home' for both of us.
Though Peter never lived there he would use it whether I was
there or not as a place to relax, to read, to listen to his
records—Beethoven, Bach, Mahler—in peace, never a characteristic of the Wright household. In most practical ways he had,
I think, opted out of his responsibilities there: Helena ruled the
roost, arranged for (rather than lived with) the four boys, so that
they were rarely either underfoot or available for Peter to make a
real relationship with them. But—as he said to me once (the
only time we touched on his relationship with Helena), 'She and

I are going in the same direction.' Her way was not his way, but the goal was the same—the service of other people.

We were, I think, Peter and I, both lonely. For me Peter was a guru, introducing me gradually to a world of culture and ideas which we could share. Before this I had absorbed alone the impact of Italian art, for example, or the discovery of D. H. Lawrence ('disgusting' to my family). Now Peter and I could giggle at Cortot's tuneless humming as he played the opening bars of Beethoven's 'Moonlight Sonata' and we could share poetry or philosophy with open minds never, obviously at least, teacher and taught (uninformed) as it had always in the past been for me. Clearly, however, Peter was a born teacher and should have had much more opportunity to teach than the closed world of the medical profession ever allowed this missionary, returned too late to the rat-race and out of step. Where his money came from I do not know and did not ask; he must have earned very little. Helena was obviously earning a lot from her practice and had inherited some and said she possessed a 'guardian angel', but I cannot imagine Peter living on her money. I just do not know.

Since their teens the Wright boys had been aware that their father had women friends, but his relationship with Marjorie was a more significant one than the others.

For Peter, perhaps I was in part the daughter he had never had, an undeveloped personality whose horizons he could widen, and he did. Together, often with Freda Bromhead, we explored Christian socialism, Marx, Freud, Adler, Jung. And gradually, sometimes with Beric, sometimes he and I alone, we spent most of our holidays together, often abroad—Brittany, Austria, Germany, where we noticed with horror that '*Heil Hitler*' was replacing '*Grüss Gott*'. And we eventually looked for a weekend cottage, found Shelley House in Marlow and spent with Freda and other friends regular weekends there.

Personal communication to the author—29.4.81

At Shelley House Freda Bromhead encouraged Peter's latent talent for cooking.

We used to cook at the cottage at weekends and gradually got together a *batterie de cuisine*, aiming rather at *haute cuisine*, *suprême de volaille*, etc., and collected recipes. Peter had to be restrained from dropping knives and things when they were finished with as he was apt to do in the operating theatre.

Personal communication to the author—14.1.81

Marjorie Silcock passed out of Peter's intimate life after the war. He had helped and encouraged her to become a medical student, and in 1947 she qualified in medicine. In her first hospital job she fell in love with a charge nurse, Edgar Myers, who later became a psychiatric social worker, and married him shortly afterwards. Her contacts with the Wright family and her friendship with Freda persisted throughout the rest of her life.

During the years in London Helena had cultivated her own friendships—perhaps the reason for Peter's loneliness. Her weekends were often spent with Tom Hill, an increasingly successful architect, and their long relationship survived many years of quarrels and differences. Helena has herself described Tom as 'arrogant, egocentric and selfish'. She believed she 'was the only person who mattered in his life,' although there is little doubt that he often took advantage of her and abused her generosity. He and Helena spent many holidays together, perhaps Whitsun in Finland or a week climbing in Skye. She often stayed in his house, Valewood, near Haslemere, and later shared with him the expenses of Daneway, a house at Sapperton near Cirencester until he married at the age of sixty-two a girl many years his junior. Mary Ainslie has described a visit to Tom and Helena there:

> It was a most beautiful house with mosaics all the way up the pillars. Tom had no idea of domesticity or getting food in. He was eccentric and not very practical, but she [Helena] could buy the food. She disliked housework so always said she was not domesticated, but she could manage very well if she was left with no one to do it for her.
>
> Personal communication to the author—7.4.82

Helena's relationship with Bruce McFarlane was more harmonious, and there is reason to suppose that Bruce was the person who mattered most to *her*. After their meeting in All Souls he became an accepted member of her family, unlike Tom whom they all disliked, and he always spent Christmas with them. Bruce was the only child of conventional Scottish parents whom he hated, according to Helena.

As senior fellow of Magdalen, he lived in the college for thirty years, an outstanding mediaeval historian and scholar of international repute who was elected to the British Academy and the Society of Antiquaries. Helena maintained that her friends had to be more intelligent and cleverer than herself and Bruce satisfied this criterion. The year he died he had been made Reader in History at Oxford, having turned down a chair of great distinction elsewhere. He was an inspiring teacher who attracted large audiences, a perfectionist with a streak of melancholy which Helena could often dispel. Bruce McFarlane was interested in Romanesque churches and Helena and he drove all over France together, with Helena in the role of pupil. According to Helena, Peter offered no objections and Helena encouraged him to take his women friends on his holidays. Her own holidays with Bruce or Tom were limited to term times, while school holidays were dutifully kept for her children. She believed marriage was a 'social responsibility' but said, 'I was prepared to be unconventional.' She was able to convince herself that it helped her sons to have parents with unorthodox views. She referred to one of Peter's friends as 'the other woman in his life'.

Helena used to tell her patients that a person who was capable of two or more relationships had 'a rich personality'. When a patient complained she had found that her husband had a mistress, Helena explained that in her view the 'injured' wife should congratulate the husband, and anyway not give him the satisfaction of knowing she minded. That could only boost his ego.

Helena maintained that she would not have been at all upset herself to find *her* husband engaged in multiple sexual relationships. Nor could she share the resentment of women who after marriage found that their husbands were bisexual. These men felt guilty and had been unwilling to tell their wives the facts. Among Helena's patients a number of women expressed their distress at the discovery, but to Helena bisexuality was perfectly acceptable, and she found it difficult to help any woman who was not sympathetic to the 'natural tendencies' of her partner. In her view no woman had a right to the whole sexual valency of the man she had married. 'What are you losing,' she would ask, 'by your husband's extra richness? After all, you are the only *woman* to whom he responds sexually.'

Helena had a number of homosexual friends, as well as some who were bisexual. She was, of course, years ahead of her time in her attitude to homosexuality, and certainly did not condemn sexual practices between individuals of the same sex, which was, it should be remembered, as far as men were concerned, a criminal offence at that time. She believed fervently that everyone should make the best use of his or her sexual gifts, and that the sex life of every human being was a private affair. The only public relationship she would countenance was marriage.

Bruce and Helena wrote to one another two or three times a week. Thus:

> Most precious and beloved,
>
> The family is out exercising its and the dog's muscles in Hyde Park and I have done what clothes-washing is bearable today, so here is peace . . . and I can contemplate the riches of your two letters.
>
> The first deduction and comfort seems to be that from your point of view my recent misery about you was unnecessary—for that my heart glows again happily. The second that you made a convincing description of yourself drowned by activities, and with that I send you much understanding sympathy. The third thought is a speculation: when two people are engrossed with one another mentally, spiritually (do you allow the word?) and also sexually and emotionally, their behaviour in expressing the relationship seems nearly always to be similar in detail and in warmth, but when the sexual–physical becomes calmer the essential differences in the two personalities emerge and may cause unfounded sorrow? e.g. You seem to express yourself more naturally now by waiting until life gives you a good space of time and peace in which you can write one of your gorgeous letters. You don't feel cold and unloving and unloved on silent days while I, whether feeling sexual or not, crave a frequent, however short, communication from you which can be seen and handled and vividly felt. I don't value the long letters any less, but where you really don't enjoy scraps I do. So let's compromise: you needn't feel you must wait for time for a long letter, but realise however much you may despise my feminine-ness that any script from you is precious. I miss not knowing what you do every day in detail. And I will try to believe that you *do* like a short letter now and then between long ones. What do you say? Please answer. It's so glorious to feel inwardly happy about us, and the days are so dank and hollow when a long silence from you is in progress.

I'm not conscious of feeling distant at any time, but that impression may be caused by the differences in self-value you and I put upon ourselves. You honestly do value yourself highly (and rightly I think). You know your value to me beyond possibility of doubting. Whereas I value myself very little; it truly is a mystery to me why anybody should find me valuable, and I'm constantly apprehensive of being a bore to you. You let me bore you for years by my descriptions etc., in silence, and I had to force your reaction out of you more or less by chance. You can easily imagine how a fear can spread outwards from an experience like that, can't you? I'd so much prefer you to tell me as sharply as you feel every time I do bore you, but I have little hope! . . .

Your loving
Helena
HRW to KBMcF—'Home', 13.12.42

After Tom's marriage, for seven years Helena rented the Dower House at Stonor, a small farmhouse on Lord Camoys' estate where she and Bruce shared the expenses. According to Helena:

> There we had our apprenticeship and I watched how quickly Bruce learnt things. He was quite fierce, but we were so independent. Then he had to put up with me at Quainton.
> Personal communication to the author—21.7.80

In 1962 Helena bought Brudenell House, previously the Quainton Rectory, near Aylesbury, from the Church Commissioners for £6,500. It was a Grade II listed building and the sixtieth house she had looked at in the area. Quainton fulfilled one particular requirement —it was equidistant between Oxford and London, so that Bruce could reach it easily from Oxford and they could share their weekends there.

The rectors of Quainton had probably occupied the original building since the thirteenth century. During his incumbency (1507–22) George Brudenell made major alterations to the mediaeval hall, and subsequent rectors had added further rooms. It was much too large for twentieth-century rectors to maintain and the last incumbent had ceased to make any effort to do so. When Helena took it over it was in extremely bad repair. Together she and Bruce restored the house and with her help Bruce furnished it with exquisite antique furniture. The house and garden became a haven of immense beauty.

The relationship between Helena and Bruce McFarlane was an unusual one. When he died he left all his possessions to Helena, making her husband his executor. He dedicated his important book, *John Wycliffe and the Beginnings of English Non-Conformity* (1952) 'To Helena for whom the book was written'. Both Helena and he had other relationships, but their lives were central to one another. After the move to Quainton Helena referred to Bruce as 'my tenant', and such letters from him as are available consist largely of discussions —sometimes on the querulous side—regarding the maintenance of the Rectory. The intimacy which existed between Helena and her 'tenant' was accepted as such not only by her family and friends, but even by her secretary Joan Leslie. That Bruce could also wound her emotionally is clear from a letter she wrote from Lake Garda, where she went every year to visit her friend Ceril (Princess) Birabongse, and to paint her many water-colours.

Some misunderstanding or unhappiness had evidently passed between Bruce and Helena before her departure from England, concerning the purchase of property after leaving Stonor.

10.45 a.m. 80°F in the Garden Room, a grey and stuffy day. Darling, having lived with you for thirty years, I have at last learned to say nothing in self defence. You hold your opinions as if cast in concrete . . . If there had been more time for thought I might have foreseen that such an apparent sudden change of decision over a question that had already become rather tiresome would have produced one of your quirks of behaviour which I know well. We will be doing something, cooking, looking for a hotel, anything frustrating and you will suddenly give up, saying in an enraged, imperious voice 'I'm not going to . . . whatever it is' and figuratively flounce off. The difficulty isn't ever anything real, like trying to climb a palm tree with slippery shoes, but apparently the obstacles suddenly seem not worth the effort. Luckily this doesn't happen in your work . . . there obstacles are a stimulus, as far as I know, you don't give up until you are satisfied that no more is possible at the moment. So I sorrowfully decide that my behaviour was impulsive, clumsy and tactless.

There's another aspect which is stinging me into sorrow day and night, in spite of the absorbing beauty of this place and the extraordinary kindness of Ceril and Bruno, and that is the revelation, like the lightning shaft of death flashing through me, that you don't regard our being together as of primary importance as I do. I find I had thought, without distinctly recognising it, that we had by now our foundations on rock immovable in this life, now it seems that is not so. Where are we? . . . Presumably I still have some value for you. What is it? . . .

Ceril sends warm greetings. To you I continue, as always, to send all the love you will accept. I hope my absence is allowing you to do rewarding work.

Your loving
Helena

HRW to KBMcF—Punta Campagnola, 21.1.61

I first went to Quainton with Helena on a wet and windy day in 1981. 'I feel at peace as soon as I get here,' she said. We were in her bedroom with its large bay window looking over the garden she loved to the hills beyond Quainton village. She slept in her father's marquetry bed from his Paris flat, and on the walls were her own delicate water-colours, which she had painted in Sicily and in Italy, and one of the view from Valewood where she and Tom had painted during the war. There was a water-colour of a stallion by her friend 'Billy' Leach whose paintings also adorned her rooms in London, and the nude which Eric Gill had given her.

Bruce had died of a stroke in 1966. On a picnic excursion together, Helena, wondering why he had not returned to the car after lunch, found him unconscious a few yards from the road, and he died in hospital without regaining consciousness. His presence had left a permanent mark on the house at Quainton. His library still held his books in four enormous bookcases, and one of the two dining-rooms contained the chairs and desk from his Magdalen study. The long sofa in the bay window of his study still looked over the lawn. Without Bruce's financial support the house became a liability and Helena eventually sold it to Beric, retaining a life interest herself. Quainton was 'home' to her for twenty years and she intended, she told me, to die there.

During the Second World War, Helena continued her usual work but with added commitments as a member of the medical committee of the FPA. She was immediately concerned about the women who were joining the armed forces. They must be protected from the hazards of pregnancy, and she took it upon herself as secretary of the

FPA Medical Sub-Committee, to try to convince the powers at the War Office of this need. Helena wanted the FPA to provide a complete contraception service for all serving women, and to train the army's medical officers in the technique. At the War Office an official she interviewed flatly refused the offer and seemed surprised to think young service women had any need of such help. As a compromise Helena offered to house pregnant service women in her home. A number of girls eventually turned up at Randolph Crescent, where they helped in the house for a reasonable wage. Helena arranged for the delivery of their babies and if necessary found nurseries afterwards or organised an adoption.

Peter joined the Emergency Medical Service and at St Margaret's Hospital at Epping he and his colleagues transformed what had been an old workhouse into a good general hospital where some of the London Hospital medical students were trained. In 1940 he returned to Randolph Crescent, from where he used to shuttle between St Margaret's Hospital, Epping, and Queen Mary's Hospital, Stratford. He continued to work as well at the French Hospital and also took on the surgery at Edenbridge and Erith Cottage Hospitals in Kent.

Much of his energy and time was taken up with arguments with bureaucrats, about, for instance, his petrol allocation for emergency visits in his Buick to his hospitals. The war was a difficult time for him, and his son Beric Wright noticed that it aged his father considerably. As Freda Bromhead has put it:

> Often when Peter was operating at one hospital a message would come asking him to go on to another because of some emergency, instead of coming home. He had no registrars, no one he could trust to take instructions on the telephone and would come home perhaps at 2 o'clock in the morning during the London Blitz.
>
> Personal communication to the author—20.1.81

Freda used to keep the one rationed bottle of whisky a month with which to revive him on these occasions.

Freda Bromhead left Randolph Crescent after the war and for a period the domestic situation there became somewhat precarious, until the arrival of one Frederika in 1947 who, in Helena's words, was 'a gift from Heaven or rather Tom Hill. She cooked as well as they do at the Ritz.' Frederika had applied to Tom for the job of housekeeper in his London house in Cliveden Place, and Tom asked Helena to come and vet this Mrs Waldburgh, as he was not sure if he wanted someone so obviously a lady. It turned out that 'the lady' did not want the job anyway—she had been deterred by the pictures of nude boys on the marble wall in Tom's hall—but Helena liked her on sight and had told Tom he should take her. However, the following day Frederika arrived at Randolph Crescent to tell her that she would rather work for her than for Mr Hill, and would be coming to Randolph Crescent. This suited Helena very well and thereafter peace reigned in the Wright household for the next six and a half years. Frederika was the American widow of an Austrian diplomat. After his death she had come to visit her sister in London, thought she would like to stay there, but could only get a work permit if she would do housework or hospital work. She chose the former.

She arrived at Randolph Crescent to find the departing servants had left her some fish in the frying pan on the stove but almost nothing in the store cupboard and all Helena's rations used up. Soon after this Helena noticed a letter addressed to Countess von Waldburgh zu Wolfegg und Waldsee—which turned out to be the names of the castles owned by her late husband the Count. After that Frederika used to hear the boys shouting, 'Where's the Countess?' though Helena paid no attention to titles—she was much more impressed by the diamonds Frederika wore when going off duty to a party.

There were fifty-six stairs to Frederika's room at the top of the house in Randolph Crescent. She found she could not manage all the housework for such a large establishment, and persuaded Helena to let her send for two girls from her village, omitting to mention that they had been looking after her own house in Austria where her husband had been king, so to speak, of three castles. Two Tyrolean peasants, Anni and Senzi, arrived and also, with Helena's permission, Frederika's dog. Frederika was paid £5 a week, which in those days she considered good money. Helena was generous and allowed her £20 a week housekeeping money but she could be exacting, and would send Frederika off on her bicycle all over London to get food she wanted which was out of season. On one occasion Frederika's £20 housekeeping money was stolen from her purse in the market, which Olive deducted from poor Frederika's wages.

Frederika liked Helena, although 'she was not a person one got fond of', but was less impressed with Peter whom she thought a weak character. Anni and Senzi used to listen on one of the five telephone extensions to his 'flirtatious conversations' with nurses and other girl-friends, and were intrigued by the fact that when the boys' girl-friends came to stay, they sometimes did not sleep in their own beds. Frederika reported when I met her later that Olive Stewart adored Peter, but thought Helena did not treat him as well as she might.

Frederika described Helena to me as being:

> Very strong-minded and stable. She was the man of the family. Mr Wright had his yacht and his girls. Helena had no jealousy and no burning affection either for her husband. She smoked a lot when ordering the meals and was quite happy if a Duke and Duchess visited me in the kitchen.
>
> Personal communication to the author—1.10.82

The Countess von Waldburgh zu Wolfegg stayed with the Wrights for nearly seven years, and Helena had, apparently, assumed she would be with them for ever. However, eventually Frederika decided to sell her Austrian property and invest in a London home of her own. She went back to Austria and returned to England, bringing with her in her car many of the antiques her husband had left her. I found her living in North London, surrounded by treasures from her husband's castle. Among this collection, she had chosen to adorn her hall with the framed certificate of the Institute of Advanced Motorists dated 23 June 1960, evidence that she had passed the advanced test at the age of sixty-five. It was probably one of her most cherished possessions. At eighty-seven, when I first met her, she was still pretty and elegant, and still grateful to Helena for letting her have her dog at Randolph Crescent. Senzi and Anni, whom she called 'my girls', had not returned to their native Tyrol either, but had both married in England. From them she had learnt of Helena's death.

Frederika kept a diary all the time she lived with the Wrights. The Countess seems to have been regarded as a member of the family and would sometimes join them for the evening meal on a special social occasion. The three younger boys were still periodically at home but Beric was by then married.

While still a student in 1953 Michael married his first wife, Margaret, who herself became a doctor and later a specialist in child psychiatry. The marriage broke up and he later married Candida Verity, Tom Hill's great-niece, whom he had met at Tom's memorial service in 1968. Candida had known Helena from the days when Helena and her much loved uncle had shared Daneway. Frederika did not go to Michael's first wedding but she remembered attending Christopher's marriage to Daphne Hall in 1951, which took place at the church, since rebuilt, in Warwick Avenue near the Wrights' home. She had helped with the preparations for the reception. She thought Christopher was his mother's favourite and that he was extremely good-looking: 'The girls were mad about him.' After the marriage he and his wife lived at the top of his parents' house in the old nurseries. 'I shall never leave you, Mummy,' he had told his mother. Nor did he, remaining at Randolph Crescent until his death. Helena subsequently confirmed his charm with women. 'The girls all fell around him, although he was not particularly physical. Every time he came on leave in the war he brought a different girl with him.' Helena found one girl crying in the hall because he had gone out without her. 'Silly girl' was all Christopher said when his mother reproached him.

Christopher had met Daphne Hall in 1947, when he was stationed at Trincomalee. Her father was a tea-planter and when he was on leave Christopher had inveigled out of her mother an invitation to a dance at the estate in Kandy. He had found her daughter Daphne a welcome relief from the boredom of monitoring the movements of aircraft on the east coast of Ceylon. Their marriage lasted ten years until Daphne divorced Christopher in 1961, and during this time she had three miscarriages and two premature girls who lived only a few hours. This was a sad blow for Helena who longed for granddaughters. Daphne was still fond of Christopher when she divorced him but she did not approve of his financial enterprises—she has since admitted that she might have remarried him 'if things had been different'. Meanwhile he continued to live at Randolph Crescent. Daphne described him to me as 'a perennial bachelor, a man who was quick-witted and wanted fun'. Winters were for skiing and summers for sailing. His brother Beric called him:

> A shrewd cookie, incredibly attractive, charismatic, with enormous gifts which he never used; he could draw, he had a musical ear and he was charming, good-looking and a polymath.
> Personal communication to the author—26.11.80

He had inherited both the good and bad characteristics of his Lowenfeld grandfather, his charm, his Rolls-Royce mentality, his attitude to women, his love of antiques and the good things of life. Helena recognised a similarity in their horoscopes.

Christopher believed in his grandfather's axiom: buy cheap and sell dear, but Henry Lowenfeld had had a broader outlook and was shrewder and infinitely more successful than Christopher, though he could be devious on occasion, as when, it is reported, lunching in a country inn Henry once noticed on the floor a rug which he recognised as valuable. He spilt a bottle of wine on it, apologised profusely, offered the landlord a sum well below the market value in recompense, rolled up the rug and left with it under his arm.

Helena liked Daphne and Daphne liked Helena, but she found Helena an enigma, a paradoxical mixture of the unconventional and the orthodox, the former characteristic doubtless inherited from her father, the latter from her mother. For instance, Helena had fitted Daphne with a contraceptive cap but was irked when Christopher and Daphne openly shared a bedroom before their marriage while staying with Tom and Helena at Daneway. Helena explained that this might offend the domestics without apparently considering that her own position in Tom's house could be regarded as anomalous. After their divorce Daphne drifted away from the Wrights and again married a man who died suddenly and tragically. When Christopher died she resumed her links with Helena and Peter and, particularly, endeared herself to Helena, who still looked on Daphne as a daughter-in-law, and acted like a grandmother to the adopted children of her second marriage.

Christopher had disappointed his mother even before he was born. It had taken five menstrual cycles for her to conceive after she had decided to have her second child, and then the baby turned out to be another boy. As a toddler, he was often disobedient and in China he caught mumps from her by going into her room when expressly forbidden to do so. Beric remembered his young brother as an unhappy whining child, while Helena recalled that he was a self-sufficient independent little boy who would always try to go it alone.

He was apparently quite happy in England until he was taken away, with Beric, from their school in Bembridge. From then on things went wrong for him at all his schools except Millfield; then came the fiascos in the services. After the war he engaged in various doubtful commercial activities and in 1949, he embarked on the disastrous 'crabs and lobsters' project. The idea behind 'crabs and lobsters' was to collect them in the summer off the west coast of Ireland, store them alive and sell them out of season at an inflated price. With his brother Michael, Christopher set about acquiring a boat and a crew and arranged to transfer the crabs and lobsters to a salt-water pond he had found in the

Hampshire village where Peter now kept his boat on the Hamble. Before their marriage Daphne and Christopher lived on this boat, and if Peter wanted to use it himself they moved to a caravan behind the boat-house.

Christopher signed eleven different forms in connection with the mortgage, which Peter and Helena guaranteed, on the new boat, the *Vidra*, which cost over £3,000. The tidal water in the pond in Hampshire where the lobsters were stored proved inadequate and moreover was polluted by Fawley refinery. Even the boat was unsatisfactory. The enterprise proved a disaster, and was liquidated.

Helena, who could never deny Christopher anything and had indulged him since his birth, was left to pick up the debts. All her Lowenfeld inheritance disappeared when she broke the trust, initially set up for Alice Quicke and her dependants, to help Christopher. She and Peter lost their life insurances and were obliged to realise other assets. As Helena said:

> Peter and I were real fools. It was one of our tragedies that we allowed Christopher to fleece us. But so it was. Christopher could not succeed in any business because he was not thorough enough. He and Michael spent weeks together in very difficult circumstances but he hadn't enough experience. Christopher could drive anything but he was totally unintellectual. His joint motor business with Michael followed the lines of crabs and lobsters.
>
> Personal communication to the author—17.2.81

After this nothing went right for Christopher. Frederika thought him 'deranged'. His life was in ruins, his marriage broken, his girl-friends vanished and a soothsayer had foretold his death. He had debts of over £15,000 and had come, in Beric's words, 'to the end of the line'. Adrian's last recollection of Christopher was seeing him standing dejectedly outside Randolph Crescent, while Helena drove off for the weekend with the words, 'He'll be all right.' She did not realise how near was the final disaster. She could see he was depressed and hoped to help him by involving him in her major interest, extra-sensory perception (ESP) and experience of the 'Fourth Dimension' (4D). She found that Christopher had strong ESP and she encouraged his contact with a medium, Alexander, a young man about his own age who had his own 'control' and could readily enter into a trance. Together with Alexander, Helena and Christopher held seances in their home with four or five other people who came weekly or fortnightly 'to develop whatever capacities each brought of their ESP possibilities'. According to Helena, Christopher with Alexander's help got in touch with an unknown character on the other side called John. 'So from your point of view thoroughly phoney, you think it all nonsense,' she told me—although I had not said so—and continued, 'That doesn't make any difference. It's real to me.'

It may also have been real to Christopher but it was not enough for him. Eventually he persuaded his mother to help him increase his trance potential with LSD. At that time the drug was coming into psychiatric use to shorten the process of psychoanalysis. Under its influence patients could be guided more quickly through their past lives and would then talk readily about their early experiences, so helping the analyst to identify the individual's difficulties. Christopher had heard about this but he wanted nothing to do with the past; it was the present and the future that interested him. Here was a chance for him to exploit his newly found extra-sensory powers. 'We don't need doctors,' he told his mother. 'We can do it without them. You write the prescription.' Helena declined, but 'like a short-sighted idiot I agreed to Christopher's request to get a psychiatrist who had used the drug successfully for a few of my patients to let Christopher have the LSD.' It was another example of Helena's innate ability to get whatever she wanted. It turned out to be totally disastrous.

Helena had asked her psychiatrist colleague to accept the responsibility and with the medium, Alexander, Christopher paid several visits to her. The psychiatrist gave them a room to themselves but did not attend the sessions which followed the taking of the dose of LSD. In Christopher's words, this gave them 'the most extraordinary experiences. Why don't you come and share them?' he asked his mother. Helena refused but she was totally convinced that to Christopher the experiences were real. He had been able, for instance, she believed, to leave his body one night when he found himself above the roof of the house, and he could make contact with people 'on the other side'. 'His business ability was not real but there was no doubt or swindling about his 4D.'

On the fatal day, 6 September 1962, Alexander noticed during an LSD session that Christopher was suddenly having difficulty in breathing, and he then collapsed. Alexander called the psychiatrist, but to no avail. An oxygen cylinder proved to be empty and there was no resuscitation equipment to hand. Christopher was dead on arrival by ambulance at the Middlesex Hospital. Peter broke the news to Helena on the telephone: 'Something dreadful has happened . . .'

Though the psychiatrist had given both Christopher and Alexander an antidote (chlorpromazine) to LSD which should have been taken at the end of each session to arrest the action of the drug, it transpired that Christopher had omitted to take this. At the autopsy he was found to have a displacement of his heart and, following an inquest held on 11 September and 13 November 1962, the coroner brought in a verdict of 'Accidental death from ventricular fibrillation due to Lysergic Acid Diethylamide'.

It was already known that Christopher had a displacement of the heart but this had caused no previous symptoms. His death was the first reported in the United Kingdom from LSD, and the assumption was made that Christopher's sensitivity to the drug had led to fatal alteration of the heart rhythm. The psychiatrist escaped criticism from the public but not from Helena, who regarded her colleague as culpable in not checking that Christopher had actually taken the antidote.

> The whole thing was so painful . . . I had nothing more to do with her, and couldn't trust myself to speak to her again because I felt it was so monstrous.

It wounded Helena terribly to find that Christopher had deceived her:

> He took lying very easily in his stride. I think it would be fair to say he treated me dishonestly because he never told me he did not take the antidote. He took the LSD with my permission as the only way of getting it. He had everything he wanted. His parents were his victims but I don't think he voluntarily hoodwinked us. Every time he came up with a proposition he completely believed in it himself.
>
> Personal communication to the author—3.2.81

Alexander later reported that while in the psychiatrist's room he saw two people in 4D fighting for Christopher after the tragedy had occurred. Helena told me that on the same evening of Christopher's death she was in the room in which the seances at Randolph Crescent had been held, when she heard a little voice which could only have been Christopher's say, 'I'm so sorry, Mummy.' This is how she described the incident to me:

You can never get over it but I have assimilated it by continuing contact with Christopher, hearing how he has taken it and what he has been doing since . . . Christopher was lost accidentally and quite unnecessarily. He was not lost from other people's point of view. The two people whom Alexander saw fighting for him kept hold of him and kept him under their care. One of them was this John who took this responsibility with me [Helena] and has taken the whole charge of Christopher's development . . . The key when Christopher said, 'I'm so sorry, Mummy', was that now he could see himself in quite a different way. He went over to the other side in very bad shape. He had behaved badly according to our rules.

There are some people who simply cannot give credence to what happens after death and the vast majority of unbelievers don't know they are dead. It's the only thing that's left of hell. They sit in a little grey cloud and don't believe they're there. Christopher's job is to go to this nasty region, where the materialists are sitting out aeons of time, where it's dank and smelly. He finds it very tiring but John keeps him there because he needs the discipline.

Personal communication to the author—18.2.81

Helena's reaction to Christopher's death is further revealed in a letter she wrote to Bruce McFarlane five days later:

Darling, I must thank you for being so kind, so delicately kind to me at the weekend. I was afraid that you might want me even less than usual as I was in a state of badly concealed misery. Instead you gave me warm comfort. I returned to London better able to endure.

The sharp sting of loss is getting slightly less and there's so much to do that even memories are sometimes forced into the background. The funeral is on Thursday morning—meaningless but unavoidable . . .

HRW to KBMcF—11.9.62

She ended with the words, 'So much love and gratitude, Your Helena,' but it is a measure of her ability to keep her life in strict compartments that the second part of this letter at a time of terrible distress is concerned with the description of a house that she thought it might suit her to buy and share with Bruce.

Helena succeeded in rationalising Christopher's death. When I asked her if she was any happier now about the tragedy, she replied:

> Absolutely happy and so is he. He has saved several people and John is pleased with him. Christopher was the first one of our group. Since then a number of people have joined it—we call it being rescued, but my time in using my ESP is strictly limited by what they can give.
>
> Personal communication to the author—18.2.81

She was referring to contact in the Fourth Dimension with Bruce and Peter after their deaths, with whom at the end of her life she held regular conversations and believed they replied.

I once asked her if any of her remarks to me were to be regarded as confidential, to which she answered:

> What I have told you is entirely for you to use as you wish . . . From my point of view it is as real as the biscuits on this plate. The chocolate biscuit is brown, the other pale yellow. You've got to see it as a logical fact and that I'm responsible—not you. You can't be responsible for anything that is not your own experience. It is a vital part of my history and I would go further. As the 4D experience is so real to me I think the more people who know about it the better. Let them know. It doesn't matter what they think, or what their ideas are. Among your general public there'll be a few who'll catch on and say: 'Of course, that's what happens to me.' So very slowly it grows but by my method and your method it only grows honestly . . . Experience must be individual. It's a tortuous development . . . because you don't know what you are working on. That's my experience in the past and it is still going on now.
>
> Personal communication to the author—26.2.81

[11]

Wider Fields

The National Birth Control Association became the Family Planning Association in May 1939, at what Dr C. P. Blacker has described as an 'agitated' Extraordinary General Meeting. At that time the falling birth rate was causing public anxiety and according to Dr Blacker the name of the NBCA was changed as a result of the depopulation scare. The NBCA objectives were therefore revised, and under its new name the FPA was pledged henceforth to work for facilities which would enable married women either to space their families or to limit them in order to avoid ill health and poverty. The FPA was to establish centres which could offer advice on sterility, minor gynaecological ailments and the psychological difficulties within marriage. The Association was at pains to explain that it was not anti-baby, only anti too many babies for women who already had all they could look after.

Within four months the Second World War broke out. FPA activity declined and the promised provision of more clinics came to a halt. Helena continued to try to get contraception services organised by the FPA as a right for all women in the forces, but the head of the ATS medical services, Dr Letitia Fairfield, a Catholic, was opposed to birth control. Her successor, in 1942, Dr (later Dame) Albertine Winner, though co-operative, was averse to publicity and unsympathetic to the idea of giving advice to the unmarried girls who comprised a majority in the force. All women in the services were entitled to see a woman doctor if they so wished, but with only a limited number of women doctors available many girls were sent to civilian doctors who, if asked, gave what contraceptive advice they could.

Other difficulties arose from a shortage of rubber, which threatened the supply of diaphragms. Rubber was required for the free-issue condoms supplied under government contract to men in the armed forces with the object of preventing venereal disease. Married, and certainly unmarried, women were in danger of losing out until a supply of rubber sheeting destined for French hotel bathrooms came to hand. This rubber had a marbled appearance and the diaphragms which the London Rubber Company was then able to manufacture looked somewhat bizarre. Some women who kept them as souvenirs were reportedly later heard to refer to them as 'Helenas'.

More significantly, from Helena's point of view, the war prevented international contacts between those countries which already had organised family planning associations—the USA, Holland, Sweden and the United Kingdom. She had become increasingly interested in the international aspect and in 1930 had attended a conference in Zurich on International Birth Control where with Dr C. P. Blacker she was a United Kingdom delegate. In Zurich Helena had met Margaret Sanger who had organised the First World Population Conference in Geneva three years previously, Dr Abraham Stone, also from the USA, Professor Hans Harmsen of Germany's family planning movement, and Elise Ottesen-Jensen, the Scandinavian social reformer whose main interest lay in sex education in schools. These pioneers were later to form the nucleus of a worldwide international movement.

After the war Helena was disappointed to find a lack of international interest on the part of the British FPA, largely due to the attitude of Lady Denman who, in spite of being a friend of Margaret Sanger's, had, according to Helena, 'no world feeling', though Helena admired her other qualities which made her 'the perfect Chairman'. Instead the FPA turned its attention to a new interest, sub-fertility, and made little attempt to encourage state support for future family planning services, with the result that no provision for this was made in the National Health Service Act of 1946. Until then the major achievements of the FPA had been largely due to Helena Wright, but after the passing of the Act the FPA concentrated on providing more clinics itself and on extending its facilities, including pregnancy diagnosis in its own laboratory. It was to run most of the birth control clinics in Britain for over forty years until April 1974, when comprehensive family planning advice services became the responsibility of the new NHS authorities and the FPA handed over more than a thousand clinics.

Helena disapproved throughout of what she called the FPA's 'small-minded and introverted' attitude, and continued to urge it to look beyond the English Channel at what was going on in the rest of the world. Her international hopes came nearer to realisation when Elise Ottesen-Jensen organised the first International Conference on

Birth Control in Stockholm in 1946. This conference set up a committee run by Edward Griffith to arrange an international meeting in England, on 'Population and World Resources' at Cheltenham, in 1948. Edward Griffith immediately asked Helena and Beric Wright to join the organising committee. The FPA declined to be officially involved at this stage since it was busy at the time organising a conference on sub-fertility in Oxford.

At this point Margaret Sanger arrived in Europe. Before leaving the USA she had created consternation by declaring a 'moratorium on all births in Britain and other hungry countries until the economic situation is adjusted'. The press publicity that greeted her arrival in England brought further confusion. Members of the British Family Planning Association respected Mrs Sanger for her early pioneering work in America, and Helena liked and admired her, although she was already proving unduly autocratic. However, unlike Marie Stopes, Margaret Sanger could work with doctors and set out to persuade the FPA to support the coming international conference which was to be held at Cheltenham. Lady Denman did not want the skeleton services of the British FPA diverted, but the executive finally agreed to take the responsibility for the conference arrangements. To Helena's great pleasure it fell to her, with Beric's help on the small planning committee, to organise the programme. 'I was blissfully happy,' she later recalled. 'Here was the seed, the egg, the grain for an eventual world movement.'

The delegates at Cheltenham came from twenty-three countries, with Helena and Margaret Pyke representing the British FPA. Helena considered the speakers were all exceptionally good—apart from Joseph Needham, FRS, adviser to UNESCO, with some of whose views Helena disagreed—and the conference was a triumph for her and a turning-point of great importance in the international field. From then on there was a gradual but steady interest in the world movement. Helena and Margaret Pyke were mainly responsible for organising a new body, the International Committee on Planned Parenthood (ICPP). Helena was made Treasurer of the ICPP (which later became the International Planned Parenthood Federation). A part-time secretary, Helen (later Lady) Cohen, was appointed for a short while, followed by the full-time appointment of Vera (later Lady) Houghton.

Helena had interviewed Vera Houghton for the post and had told her that one of her main tasks was 'to keep the Americans happy because they had all the money'—collected by Margaret Sanger. At the time of her interview Vera Houghton was already known to Helena and Margaret Pyke as she had applied, unsuccessfully, for the job of General Secretary of the FPA, but had been turned down by Lady Denman who may have been doubtful about appointing the wife of a Labour politician, Douglas (later Lord) Houghton. Vera Houghton was an extremely successful Executive Secretary of the IPPF for ten years, and Helena has said that she doubted if the IPPF would have turned out as it did without her: 'She was the perfect choice.'

Vera Houghton found Helena 'very businesslike and financially-oriented. There were no grey areas in her; she was a business woman.' She was later on Helena's death to add to this testimonial:

> The practical businesslike qualities with which Helena Wright was endowed were particularly valuable . . . Statements of accounts and budgets were meticulously gone through and her careful stewardship made it possible for us to survive nearly two years on the initial grant of £1,200 from the Brush Foundation of the United States.
>
> Helena's ability to concentrate to the exclusion of all else on the immediate subject, whether a budget, future policy, a trainee doctor or a patient, was invaluable. It meant that she always had time to listen, to assess and then to map the way ahead.[1]

The IPPF officially came into existence on 29 November 1952 at the Third International Conference in Bombay. This conference had been Margaret Sanger's idea. After Cheltenham, India's progress had been phenomenal, and furthermore she had the power to influence other Asian countries with needs as great or greater than her own. In 1951 the First All-India Conference on family planning had been covened by Dhanvanthi Rama Rau, a former president of the All-India Women's Conference and the originator of the Family Planning Association of India. While the delegates were arriving for the conference in December 1951 Lady Rama Rau was disconcerted to receive a cable from Margaret Sanger, asking if she and her team would be prepared to hold the next international conference the following year in India. Lady Rama Rau agreed, with some reservations. In fact, the ICPP had already decided to hold the next

---

[1] *People* (1982), vol. 9, No. 2

conference in Sweden, which took place later in 1953 when the
IPPF's constitution was formulated. It had fallen to Dr C. P. Blacker
to draft the constitution. According to Helena, Dr Blacker was ideally
suited to the task, having 'the faculty of putting muddled ideas into
a common denominator'.

The Dutch in particular were outraged at Mrs Sanger's undemocra-
tic and autocratic initiative in changing the venue of the International
Conference. Although plans to hold the 1952 Conference in Bombay
went ahead, the general annoyance increased when the ICPP *News*,
which was published in America, announced that Lady Rama Rau
had *invited* the committee to hold the conference in India. Fourteen
countries were represented at Bombay by nearly five hundred delegates, and as Beryl Suitters has observed, 'India probably had more
impact on the international family planning movement than the movement had on India.'[2] For Helena the conference marked another
milestone in her life and was the beginning of her strong and lasting
friendship with Lady Rama Rau. Bombay was for her the gateway to
India, a country she came to love 'as almost my second country', and
to which she was to return seven times in all.

At the Bombay Conference in 1952 Helena spoke on the 'Technical
and Scientific Aspects of Family Planning'. The Pill was still only a
speck on the horizon, although interest was already centred on it at the
conference. Helena described all that was known of barrier and
spermicide prevention of invasion by the male sperm. She went on to
mention the preliminary work being done in England to alter the
nature of cervical mucus so that it would obstruct the passage of
sperms into the womb, and referred to American research into the
possibility of making it harder for the male sperm to penetrate the
surface of the egg. There was favourable mention by Helena of the
FPA *Approved List of Contraceptives*, and the durability of condoms,
and she concluded that, 'In the present state of knowledge—or
ignorance—a double method is the only one which has been found to
be reliable,' a conclusion that holds good today as far as the barrier
methods are concerned.

Helena hoped that a cheaper substance than rubber or plastic would
soon be available for the peoples of Asia unable or unwilling to buy
the comparatively expensive alternatives, and described how village

[2] Beryl Suitters, *Be Brave and Angry*: Chronicles of the International
Planned Parenthood Federation (1973).

midwives could be taught to make tampons of cotton or silk waste, tied round with a strong thread. The user could make these herself and keep a stock 'in any ordinary household crock'. Every night she should smear one all over with a chemical, and push it as far as it would go into the vagina.

> If intercourse takes place she leaves the ball in till about midday next day; if not she pulls it out when she gets up, and in both cases she simply burns the ball and string . . . The only foreign importation will be the chemical . . . and it is not impossible that local substitutes might be found for even that . . . As the midwives are already in natural relations with the families of the village it may well turn out that these village midwives will be the first teachers of family planning in the vast village population of India.

Helena ended her address with a reference to the safe period, concluding that 'in practice causes of failure are sooner or later found to be unavoidable'. Her final hope was that 'this conference will succeed in the setting up of organisations and methods that will give intelligent control to world population and at the same time enormously increase the security and happiness of the mothers of India'.

She could not foresee the problems that India was to face in her long policy of organised population control, something Helena could not accept. Throughout her life she was a staunch supporter of the right—even duty—of every woman to control her own fertility. Long before the Cheltenham Conference population control had already become a controversial issue. The implications were well described at the Fourth IPPF Regional Conference in London in 1964:

> The reasons why persons propagate planned parenthood may be very different: one will have in mind the world's population; another will have in mind the population of a certain country in connection with the standard of living; a third one may have in mind the possibilities in life for a group like the family in relation to the demands that people make upon life, or the right of the individual to order his life in his own way also when it concerns parenthood.[3]

[3] M. Zeldenrust, Rotterdam, Holland. *Sex and Human Relations*. Proceedings of the Fourth Conference of the Region for Europe, Near East and Africa of the IPPF. London (1964).

Helena subscribed to the latter view. She used to say: 'It is the individual who must choose [how to control her own fertility]. Give women the choice and they will choose. I want to see every individual having that choice and having it freely.' At Cheltenham Joseph Needham had taken the view favoured by geneticists:

> The conscious world control of population . . . will have to be done some day by some kind of representative body, which will have to take administrative responsibility for introducing the various controls which may be necessary—the encouragement, for example, of family limitation, or the encouragement of the production of children, family allowances, and so on—geared up in a complicated way with the mechanisation of agriculture, soil conservation and so on; in fact, world planning . . . This basic optimism is extraordinarily important; we must be optimistic about the possibility of world population control . . .
>
> I admit that this is a long-term matter, and I do not fail to take account of the enormous amount of human suffering which may have to be gone through before what I look forward to is reached . . .[4]

Joan Rettie, Regional Secretary, Europe Region IPPF, has summed up the situation created at Cheltenham:

> Sex was not a subject that could easily be discussed in Britain at that time. There was and is a tendency among those anxious to overcome their own inhibitions, and those of others, to identify planned parenthood in terms of population as a suitable topic for public discussion, making it almost possible to forget that births are the result of sexual intercourse.
>
> To be fair to some of the early pioneers, who were genuinely involved in offering planned parenthood services in their own countries, they undoubtedly did not realise that by inviting the participation of neo-Malthusian theorists, unconnected with national planned parenthood associations, they would introduce neo-Malthusian politics, and change the whole basis of the aims

[4] Joseph Needham. Proceedings of the International Congress on Population and World Resources in relation to the Family. Cheltenham (1948), pp. 230–3.

agreed at the 1946 meeting, on which the IPPF might have been established in 1952.[5]

Although the neo-Malthusian members of the Eugenics Society such as Dr C. P. Blacker strongly supported Joseph Needham's speech at Cheltenham, it failed to convince Helena, which is presumably why she had described him as being the only 'difficult' speaker.[6]

At the Bombay Conference the IPPF had decided to set up regional organisations to cover South and South-East Asia, Europe and North America. Four countries in Europe—Great Britain, Sweden, Holland and West Germany— already had national organisations affiliated to the Federation. Other countries were to be offered associate membership. Although largely funded by the USA, the Federation was to be based in London, and regional offices and committees were to be established in South and South-East Asia, Europe, North America, India and London.

The constitution of the IPPF was duly ratified at the Fourth International Conference in Stockholm in 1953. Apart from reference to population control, it embodied tenets which Helena held dear, particularly an emphasis on teaching. The IPPF was among other things 'to encourage and organise the training of all appropriate professional workers such as medical and health personnel, educationalists, social and community development workers in the implementation of the objects of the Federation'. Helena had already put this to practical effect at the end of the Bombay Conference.

Her expenses in India, including her passage, had been paid by Mrs Helen Wattamull, an American who had also given the Federation one thousand dollars for research. Mrs Wattamull, who lived in Hawaii, was married to an Indian and although she had never met Helena, had decided India needed her expertise. Helena proposed to repay her by extending her visit at the end of the conference. For one week she would teach Indian gynaecologists in Bombay, and for the next two weeks she would teach village midwives. It is worth studying these three

[5] Joan Rettie, *Planned Parenthood*: A Personal View. IPPF Europe Regional Information Bulletin (April 1979), vol. 8, No. 2.

[6] Thomas Robert Malthus (1766-1835), an Anglican clergyman, held that the population increases faster than the production of food and resources required. He argued in favour of 'moral restraint' to check this increase by late marriage and coital abstinence. Neo-Malthusians accepted the Malthusian doctrine but advocated contraception in place of sexual repression.

weeks in some detail, for they were typical of her future work in India.

She stipulated that the organisers should provide her with accommodation in Bombay, and a shed was erected in one corner of the station yard. An area was partitioned off to take an examination couch and Helena's equipment. In due course thirty Indian women doctors came in groups of six for practical instruction. An Indian mother had offered to be the human model on whom Helena, accompanied by a nurse, showed the doctors—one at a time—how to fit diaphragms. When she returned to India in 1968 Helena was delighted to find one of these original pupils working in Bombay, but now in a big, well-equipped, modern clinic.

At the end of the first week Helena embarked on a two-week tour across India from Bombay to Calcutta in order to teach village midwives, on the understanding that she would stay only with Indian families. The idea of training village midwives had come from Dr Abraham Stone, who had been teaching the rhythm method in India using coloured beads. Helena, of course, had more to offer than the rhythm method in which she had little faith. Taking food and a bedding roll, in the tradition of her hero Rudyard Kipling, she took the night express to Giser in Bihar, where the Buddha had allegedly been enlightened under the peepul tree. She was met at 3 a.m. by an Indian Army officer who, again in the Kipling tradition, took her to a government rest-house. He collected her four hours later and together they set off across the plain. As they approached a little town she heard a strange booming noise—the town crier collecting her audience through a megaphone.

The town crier preceded her with his exhortations to a large colonnaded hall, where rows of doctors and midwives were seated on chairs along each side. Soon about seventy or eighty men arrived in their working clothes, some carrying their tools, and squatted in rows in the body of the hall. Helena did not know if she should address the professionals or the men on the floor. She chose the latter and, with a woman doctor as interpreter, explained in slow, simple words the basic principles of family limitation, and how this could be achieved. Eventually the blank looks on the men's faces faded and when she had finished and asked for any questions, the first man asked, 'Does the white woman mean our wives can be taught how to do this thing?' Helena could only point to her interpreter and feel the meeting had been a success. Talks for the doctors at the Lady Elgin Hospital came later.

Her next stop was Patna, the capital of Bihar. Helena was the only white woman on the train and sat on a wooden seat among the Indians 'who were so friendly I forgot I was British'. At Patna she was the guest of another Indian family, the Naths. Colonel D. P. Nath, Inspector General of Civil Hospitals in the State of Bihar, was an Edinburgh graduate whom Helena had already met during his visit to London when, with Dr Abraham Stone, they had discussed the possibility of training Indian village midwives. Helena's first task in Patna was to address a large audience of medical students, women doctors and midwives from the University Hospital, in the largest lecture theatre in the medical school, about the possibilities for the future. It was followed by a lively discussion and was for many students their first introduction by a westerner to contraceptive research and technique.

The next day, accompanied by the hospital paediatrician, the matron and another woman doctor, Helena was escorted to the village of Raj Gir where, at the local dispensary, she was introduced to the Indian district medical officer, a man. Helena had asked to meet some village women who had already had not less than five to seven children. These mothers were squatting in a semi-circle in front of the dispensary. Helena began a discussion with one of them, helped by the matron as interpreter. The ensuing conversation was not unlike ones she had held with Chinese women patients: the woman could not exactly remember how many children she had had, but only knew the number living, perhaps two or three.

'Ask her if she wants any more,' Helena demanded, and saw bewilderment on the woman's face.

'It's God who gives us children.'

'Suppose your God knew you didn't want any more?'

'Oh, how happy I would be, but it's impossible.'

'But I'm here to show you what God wants you to do when you know you needn't have any more children.'

'Teach me now!' cried the woman.

The senior medical officer, who had not been entirely pleased to be excluded, entered at this point and Helena noted the apprehension on the woman's face at his arrival, but she pointed to the village midwife, who was delighted, saying, 'Here is the one who can help you.' Asked later how she had known what to say, Helena replied that the women were not so very different from women in the poorer districts of London. Now they were receptive to the idea of asking for help from suitably trained village midwives, known locally as *dais*. She knew that midwives held a key position after each delivery and would command respect, and that she had now only to convince them of their value in teaching family planning in their own villages, including explaining the use of the cotton tampon.

During the week Helena stayed with the Naths she was introduced to a group of Mrs Nath's friends who, according to the custom of the country, were tied for life to the partner of an arranged marriage. They must obey their husbands unquestioningly and had no hope of escape because their own mothers would not accept them if they rebelled. Many could not bear the chains which bound them. 'If we were to leave the husbands we do not love and return to our own parents they would turn us out for defiant disobedience,' they said. 'And what about your own children?' asked Helena. 'Would *you* turn them out?' The women looked at her as if she had come from another world, but Helena felt she had sown a seed.

Helena's talk to the Patna Women's Council on 7 December 1952 was entitled 'How to get the best babies'. She spoke 'as a doctor with over twenty years' experience, an original member of the Executive of the British Family Planning Association, and of the International Committee for Planned Parenthood, and as mother of four sons with two grandchildren'. There were two sides of planned parenthood, teaching women how to space their families and helping couples who found it difficult to have children. She outlined the increased danger of childbirth after the fourth pregnancy, worse health in general and less resistance to disease in families where children were born too soon after one another. Helena regarded a family of three to four children as ideal in general and recommended two years between each pregnancy. She and the family planners were there for the first time to show the best of what marriage could offer. The people of Patna had splendid equipment and women doctors who could teach efficient, harmless and reasonably cheap methods of family spacing which were easy to learn. Every woman should begin now to get help and tell her friends, Helena told them.

The next stop was Calcutta airport, where Helena was to meet another Indian family, the Chaudhuris, who became permanent friends. Mr R. M. Singh, the Secretary of the Calcutta FPA, took her first to a law students' hostel where a debate on compulsory family planning was in progress. The students were evidently absorbed by the subject and then wanted a detailed report on the Bombay Conference as well as an exposition of methods of family planning. There was no need for an interpreter; they were all educated men who took in the new ideas but saw the difficulties ahead. A broadcast on All-India Radio was followed by lectures and demonstrations at the Calcutta Medical Club and the Lady Dufferin Hospital. Social activities included a party in a club where previously only men were admitted, but to which shy, well-dressed, middle-class Indian women had been invited to meet Helena. They were a new kind of audience, ready to discuss a subject that was commanding attention wherever Helena went.

Helena's desire to see New Delhi was partly due to the admiration that her friend Tom Hill, as an architect, held for Lutyens, but for herself her visit was memorable for her meeting with Indira Gandhi and Pandit Nehru. She had been introduced by her friend Isobel Cripps, the wife of Stafford Cripps, who was in Delhi at the time. Nehru's house was enormous, although they dined in a comparatively small room, and Helena and Lady Cripps were the only guests. Indira Gandhi spoke little and Helena saw her at that time only as her father's daughter. 'The feeling between them was like a radiant flame. They belonged to one another. He was entirely dependent on her and the voice in which he addressed her was different from his "thinking" voice.' To Helena he spoke as an equal about the plans for contraception in his country. He realised the Bombay Conference had been a success, recognised India's need for family planning and was sympathetic to its development on a national scale. By then family planning had already become a matter of considerable importance. The Indian parliament had just allocated 65 lakhs of rupees—about £450,000—for the national plan, and the National Planning Commission's recommendations had been fully accepted.

From now on Helena's love for India increased with every visit. She expressed her feelings in a talk to doctors during her sixth visit in 1977:

> . . . I come in great humility because I realise that it is I who will learn far more from my visit to you. Thank you all from me. I am here to talk about fertility control and family life, something I care about so passionately that I am afraid of becoming a bore . . . You can teach us so much especially in the sphere of family life, the sanctity of marriage and the care and respect for the elderly . . . This is my message to you. Hold on to your unique and in many ways your superior traditions . . .

Lady Rama Rau's daughter, Santha, a distinguished Indian writer, has left this appreciation of Helena in India:

> She seemed to feel an immediate affinity with the country and its people. My family in turn, quite simply, fell in love with Helena. Our friendship lasted thirty-one years and, because of her astonishing ability to span age differences, included four generations. If she started off in our lives as my mother's admired colleague, she soon became an important part of my sister's circle and of mine. My mother is now 89. And Helena was a marvellous friend to all of us in all our diversity of age, activities and personalities . . .
>
> . . . Then there was Helena's idea of how to spend a really satisfactory morning. What would she like to do today? I'd ask, and suggest some of the usual touristy things—the Prince of Wales Museum? The Gateway of India? A boat trip to the Elephanta Caves? Let's go to the market, she'd say . . .
>
> She liked the contrast of the plain wooden stalls of an Indian bazaar with the extravagant colours and textures of the produce piled on them—tropical fruits and vegetables, gleaming silver jewellery, brilliant silks and cottons or charming grotesque painted wooden toys . . .
>
> Helena approved the very individual attention you receive in such transactions, a small area of life where nothing is standardised . . . And she loved the great profusion of flowers, of course, but she noticed particularly the personal pride and feminine joy in the countrywomen who tucked a marigold casually into their hair, who wove roses into a little hoop to wear around a bun on the back of the head—the pleasure of women being women, a sense of decoration, an unquestioned right of anyone to the small, cheap luxuries and gaieties.
>
> But what struck me most was Helena's enthusiastic response to a kind of Indian inquisitiveness that often embarrasses foreigners. When you are engaged on an errand as prosaic as buying potatoes, in the course of the transaction your vendor may well ask you any variety of the most intrusively personal questions. Where do you live? How old are you? Are you married? How many children? Why isn't your husband with you? And so on. Far from recoiling from such impertinence, Helena not only answered the questions, but then demanded to

have her own curiosity satisfied, compelling me, for instance, to find some tactful way in Hindi of asking a baffled vegetable seller why he hadn't thought of limiting the number of his children and reducing the burden on his wife.

. . . People were Helena's most absorbing interest. India was a fascinating arena for her because Indians are incurable talkers . . . I took her once to a coffee-house where she was immediately cosy and amused . . . Looking around at the animated groups of uninhibited talkers at the tables, Helena seemed entirely at ease in the typically Indian stream of argument, scandal, anecdote, exchange of news that eddied about us. I think she liked the feeling that you can be openly interested, entertained or disapproving of the activities or remarks of the people at a neighbouring table, can, if you wish join in with your own views on any subject. Perhaps, most of all, it was this accessibility of the people that gave India so special a place in Helena's heart.

If I have made Helena seem sentimental, I have done her a disservice. Certainly she never felt any necessity to moderate her enthusiasm and appreciation, but they were always accompanied by a counterpoint of penetrating comment—tart, critical, funny, wondering—often unexpected, always original. Thinking back over the times she spent with us in India, all I really know about Helena is that I loved her. We all did. And most important, she had the extraordinary gift of knowing how to show that she loved us.[7]

The Bombay Conference was the first of a series of conferences abroad which Helena attended in connection with her official activities in the IPPF. The next highlight was the Tokyo International Conference in 1955, where by all accounts Margaret Sanger as IPPF World President was more than usually temperamental. The Japanese had until then shown little interest in contraception, relying on legal abortion and Ogino's rhythm method for fertility regulation. The demographers reported over a million successful abortions in government hospitals, which had reduced the population growth from 2 million a year to 1.3 million. The Japanese reluctantly allowed visitors into their clinics, but Helena witnessed the ten-minute operation they were doing for sterilising women with an electric cautery passed up the Fallopian tubes. After the conference she spent several days in

[7] Read at Memorial Gathering—25 May 1982, Friends Meeting House.

Thailand, where she had friends, but in teaching mainly men students she felt like 'a disciple in the wilderness'.

Apart from overseas visits, not the least of Helena's activities was the organisation of the IPPF Medical Committee. In 1934 she had been responsible for the formation of the Medical Committee of the FPA; 'Now I had to do the same thing for the world movement. I planned the IPPF Medical Committee on a Sunday in 1954 in the Cotswolds.' She presented her scheme, which was accepted, to the Federation's Executive Committee in Rome that year:

> It was the beginning of the scientific side of the Federation, and during the eight years in which I was Chairman of the Medical Committee it was fascinating to see how it spread. From modest beginnings it grew to over seventy members. We had to convince people that the growing concept was fundamentally a medical one.
>
> Personal communication to the author—28.1.80

In 1962 the structure of the main committee was changed and regional medical committees were formed under the Central Medical Committee. Helena became Chairman of the Regional Medical Committee which in 1965 was again altered to embrace four sub-committees. The shape of these committees is reflected in her letter to Sir Theodore Fox, for twenty years Editor of the *Lancet* before becoming Director of the FPA in 1964.

> . . . It is a pity that the [Regional] committee meets so seldom. When I designed the pattern of the whole IPPF Medical Committee . . . it was my hope that the new arrangement would foster self-realisation and relevant activities in the regions as distinct units. But it seems as if the regions are themselves already too large and representative meetings too expensive for this hope to have materialised to any extent. However, the regional executive medical committee does meet reasonably often and works very concentratedly, watching carefully that its activities range as widely as is practical . . .
>
> HRW to T. H. Fox—Brudenell House, 17.4.64

Rotha Peers, who had worked with Helena at Telford Road, was the first Secretary of the Medical Committee of the IPPF, and remained in the job until 1967. Mrs Peers travelled with Helena to Pakistan, Ceylon and Chile and became very fond of her. Of Helena she has said:

She was an excellent speaker and a wonderful trainer—the tops. All the overseas people admired her enormously, although she certainly didn't suffer fools gladly. When I say there were many people who loved her there were also those who didn't and who found her manner abrupt. She was too dogmatic and too matter-of-fact for some people.

> Personal communication to the author—7.6.82

Joan Rettie, who had become IPPF Regional Secretary in 1956, also admired Helena and they became friends for the rest of Helena's life. Of Helena she has said:

She was a wonderful teacher. Helena always had an open door to anyone wanting to talk about their most private life, and she could make contacts easily. She felt people must have a happy sex life and to do that they must discuss their problems and not feel ashamed. She helped very many people, even if at times she didn't always rate other people's reactions highly enough. She did not intend to hurt other people but perhaps she didn't understand other people's reactions which were sometimes different from her own. She never seemed to think that she might not be right. Perhaps there may have been some underlying doubts which she did not want to face, or even quite realise herself.

> Personal communication to the author—8.12.82

Her growing participation in international family planning left Helena less time for the British FPA, with some cooling of relations as a result. In 1952 she again urged the Association at its Annual General Meeting to widen its horizons to the international field. During the war the FPA had, of course, been unable to make overseas contacts, but Helena still regarded it as unnecessarily introspective. Lady Denman's attitude had made it difficult in this respect for Margaret Pyke who was wearing two hats: that of Secretary of the FPA, while being one of the two British representatives on the IPPF Council. The FPA also had its financial troubles at the time. It had had to move from rent-free accommodation in Eccleston Square to new offices in Sloane Street, but Miss (later Dame) Josephine Barnes, who became Chairman of the FPA Medical Committee in 1952, has agreed that the medical input of the FPA was 'rather limited' at that time: 'There was so little to offer. As far as the female section was concerned it was simply fitting diaphragms.' In Josephine Barnes's tenure of the chairmanship of the F P A Medical Committee the meetings were concerned primarily with clinic affairs, the quality control of contraceptives and whether an 'engaged' girl had to show evidence of her marriage arrangements, or if her word would be good enough.

Josephine Barnes was much younger than the other members of the Medical Committee, among them Dr Joan Malleson, Dr Margaret Jackson, and Helena. Miss Barnes supposed she had been made Chairman of the Committee 'to keep the peace among these argumentative characters'. She thought Joan Malleson 'charming, sympathetic and far-seeing. Helena was talkative, dogmatic and persuasive, but the others, including Margaret Pyke, were capable of standing up for themselves.'[8] Josephine Barnes had her own disagreements with the Committee in respect of the F P A Pregnancy Diagnosis Centre, run by the young Beric Wright, and on which the F P A relied for part of its income. She disapproved of the Association's policy of giving the result of each test, which cost twenty-five shillings, direct to the patient. She believed it should be sent initially to the patient's family doctor, claiming, 'If they [the F P A] wanted to be regarded as a professional body, they should behave professionally. In the end I won my point, after considerable argument with Margaret Pyke, but she forgave me in the end!' Some individual members still felt that married women should have as open access to F P A services as to venereal disease clinics, which were available without medical referral.

Josephine Barnes thought also that Helena should not bypass the family doctors, as she often did, in her dealings with their patients. If Helena sent a patient to see Miss Barnes in the out-patient department at University College Hospital where she was First Assistant in the Department of Obstetrics and Gynaecology, Miss Barnes would always write to the family doctor after the consultation, with a copy to Helena. Some general practitioners undoubtedly regarded Helena's practice as disreputable, although it must be remembered that medical advertising standards were in those days more strictly enforced by the General Medical Council than they are today. Helena was not *persona grata* with all doctors on this account, partly due to the notoriety her books attracted.

In the early Forties Josephine Barnes had had herself to deal with a

---

[8] Personal communication to the author—3.11.82.

minor problem when medical students at University College Hospital asked her to give them a lecture on contraception. She first learnt about the subject from what she had read in Marie Stopes's books and from hearing her lecture at Oxford when she herself was an undergraduate. There were other books available but no formal teaching was given to students. However, she was prepared to accede to the students' request, but had first to ask her professor's permission. This was granted, provided no notice about the lecture was put up in the Medical School. In her own words, 'If I had advertised my talk I think the senior staff would have turned round and sacked me.'

As late as 1954, when the IPPF had been in existence for two years, University College Hospital Medical School was the first and only one in London which, on the initiative of Professor W. C. W. Nixon, gave lectures on contraception to medical students, and in the whole country this was provided at that time only in Aberdeen, Liverpool and Edinburgh. Helena was ahead of her time in realising the importance of using the Medical Committee of the IPPF to educate doctors in the United Kingdom and overseas about birth control methods.

The Medical Committee established the medical functions of the member organisations, analysed the numbers of clinics and the services provided, including the price and types of contraceptives used in each country. It set standards for established clinics and laid down criteria for field trials. Through its Testing Sub-Committee under the chairmanship of Dr Margaret Jackson the IPPF Medical Committee ensured the quality control of contraceptives, later using the facilities provided by the FPA and University College Hospital. These findings were reported in the IPPF *Medical Handbook*, first published in 1962, which survives as the *Family Planning Handbook for Doctors*. The contents were originally overseen by Helena until Dr Ronald Kleinman was appointed editor of all IPPF medical publications in 1964.

Dr Kleinman found Helena 'quite prepared to be critical about some of the things we wrote'. This was hardly surprising since Helena was an educator, not a population controller like Margaret Sanger and other Americans. She could not, with her belief in human rights, agree with the views expressed in an early edition of the IPPF *Medical Handbook* by Dr Peter Bishop, the endocrinologist:

The problem that confronts the world is the danger of over-population by the teeming millions of uneducated people to whom the conventional methods of contraception are beyond comprehension.

To Helena population control was

> . . . one of the most dangerous and self-defeating ways of expressing our aims and intentions. Diminution of population numbers might be a result, not an aim. Our duty is to think out and to provide such improvements in education, maternal and family health and earning capacity of young people, that the careless allowing of unwanted pregnancies will become a rare mistake instead of an everyday tragedy as it is now.[9]

One of the major objectives of the IPPF was to encourage other countries to form their own organisations and appropriately Poland was the first European country to benefit from Helena's help in creating its own Family Planning Association. Early in 1957 a young Polish woman doctor, Jadwiga Beaupré, arrived at the North Kensington Clinic, on a World Health Organisation scholarship to learn about methods of contraception. She attended Helena's training course and received the customary certificate of competence. Helena had recognised immediately that she was teaching a clever and quick-witted young woman who was, incidentally, attractive and good-looking. On the last day of the course Dr Beaupré remained behind to speak to Helena and in halting German, since she could speak no English, said, 'Dr Wright, what you have done for me you must do for Poland.' The idea naturally appealed strongly to Helena, although she could see the obstacles to such a proposition in a Catholic country with a Communist government. But if there was one country she wanted to help, it was her father's homeland, and she made one stipulation only—that she should receive an official invitation from the Polish Government. This arrived through the intervention of Professor Jan Lesinski, a Warsaw gynaecologist. It was agreed that Helena's visit to Poland should follow the First Conference of the IPPF for Europe, Near East and Africa Region, which was due to take place in Berlin that autumn. Professor Lesinski and Dr Beaupré were to be the Polish delegates.

After the Berlin Conference the three arrived in Warsaw on 1

[9] Helena Wright, *Family Planning* (January 1973), vol. 21, No.4. p.89.

November 1957, to be met by two Ministry of Health officials bearing flowers. They were driven to the Hotel Bristol, occupied by the Germans during the war and barely changed from the days of Helena's youth. Now it was used only for official government entertaining and there Helena and the officials discussed the prospects for establishing an independent Family Planning Association in Poland, before Helena flew on with Dr Beaupré to Cracow which was to be the base for her teaching programme during the first week. In the next two weeks she visited three other cities, Nova Hutta, a new town outside Cracow, Bytom, the centre of the Silesian coalfields, and Posnan, before returning to Warsaw.

In every city her programme followed the same lines. Her standard lecture was translated and transcribed by a Polish gynaecologist from Helena's German script. She described the British Family Planning Association, its formation and development and the international organisation. She discussed the application of these organisations to Poland against the background of national concern for the increase in the number of legal abortions, the only recognised form of birth control, and the resulting deterioration in maternal health.

Helena had brought along her famous life-size, flesh-coloured plastic model of the female pelvis and upper thighs, complete with vaginal opening. She had designed this herself to avoid embarrassing human models when demonstrating to students the various types of diaphragms. Students would then practise on Helena's plastic replica with its front 'trap door' which when opened revealed the uterus and vaginal vault, and where the correct position of diaphragms inserted via the vagina could be seen.

This model was considered greatly superior to other models, including Margaret Sanger's. According to an English nurse Helena's model was known as 'Dr Wright's daughter'. At one time Helena thought of patenting her 'daughter', but the mirth this engendered at the Patent Office led Helena to discard the idea, since the model was evidently not in need of protection. Mrs Rettie, who accompanied Helena on many of her overseas tours, recalled comparable expressions of astonishment on the faces of customs officials. In 1982 I was amused to be shown Helena's original model, carefully preserved in a cardboard box, at the London headquarters of the IPPF—unpatented.

Helena went to Poland to teach, but she had first to establish a bridge between potential Catholic opposition and an atheist government. Her audiences were doctors, nurses and midwives, to whom Dr Beaupré would introduce Helena as a doctor from England who had a Polish father, and who had come to help Poland. Helena would then give her standard lecture and answer questions with Dr Beaupré as interpreter, repeating every sentence after her.

When she discussed the proposals for a Polish Family Planning Association with government officials, Helena advised the organisers to take the priests fully into their confidence, and to stress that uniform rules would be followed. In clinics the rhythm method only would be taught to new patients. No promise would be made that this method was infallible. As Helena explained, the rhythm method is only reliable if the woman records her daily temperature and knows by a slight rise when she is ovulating and impregnation is most likely to occur. Every woman should understand that the egg is normally released fourteen days before the next period, and that both egg and sperm have a short life. Given adequate motivation the method can be successfully applied by restricting intercourse for several days about the time of ovulation.

At the same time every clinic would be equipped with materials applicable to barrier methods of contraception. These would be offered to any woman for whom the rhythm method had failed, and who specifically asked for advice on another method. This would leave the choice to the individual. Helena's suggestions fell on the receptive ears of Eugenia Pomerskia, head of the Department of Maternal and Child Health who had issued the official invitation, and then taken an immediate and strong liking to Helena. Thereafter the Poles led the way in Eastern Europe in promoting contraception as a preferable alternative to legal abortion.

Before returning to England Helena managed, by hiring a car, to make a brief journey back to Chrzanow, which she had not visited since her father's funeral twenty-five years earlier. Now a public park, it had been taken over by the government and a plaque on the gate proclaimed the estate to be 'the gift of the People's Republic'. A few of the old villagers had heard of Helena's arrival and turned out to greet her, the last of the Chrzanow Lowenfelds.

Poland was the first of the European countries which formed family planning associations as a result of meetings between Helena and their nationals and were then able to join the IPPF. In future after nearly all regional conferences Joan Rettie arranged comparable teaching sessions.

Reporting on his visit to Poland in 1982, Julian Heddy, Director of the IPPF, Europe Region, described the situation:

> The contraceptive services in Poland work in difficult circumstances with the Government without being of the Government, and to a certain extent with the Church without being of the Church. They walk the fine line between Church and State. Many of the original founders of the Polish FPA (TRR) still remember Helena Wright with respect and affection. The diaphragm is still considered traditionally an important method of contraception. In Europe and in many developed countries, including America, you find a renaissance today of the diaphragm, whereas in Poland that tradition was unbroken, and one can trace that back to Helena Wright's particular interest in this. Many physicians in other communities are still keen on the diaphragm, having learned at the feet of Helena Wright. She was a great teacher, and everybody knew her as a great teacher.
>
> Largely through Joan Rettie's initiative, a regional training scheme was started centred on a number of teaching hospitals in London and also in Belgium and Yugoslavia . . . Through this initiative the teaching hospitals in London became increasingly interested in teaching their own students. At that time the heads of departments were very conservative about teaching contraception and establishing clinics within the hospitals, and in some way the Europe Regional scheme gave an initiative to hospitals including King's College, the Westminster and Mount Vernon hospitals.
>
> Personal communication to the author—26.11.82

In 1960 at a regional conference at The Hague, Helena received an unexpected communication from the secretary of the North Kensington Women's Welfare Centre in Telford Road, (by then an FPA clinic) which stated that as she was over-age, her appointment as Medical Officer was to be terminated. She was to receive £30 severance money—£1 for each year of service. Helena appeared unconcerned, even amused, but Mrs Rettie was so enraged that she asked Mrs Cecily Mure, the voluntary Secretary of the Walworth Clinic, who was also at The Hague at the time, if Helena could continue her teaching there. As a result Helena worked at Walworth, by then also part of the FPA, on Thursday evenings in place of her Wednesday evening sessions at

Telford Road. Later, she also taught and worked as Medical Officer at the Marie Stopes Memorial Centre.

Marie Stopes had left all her papers on her death in 1958 to the British Museum and her clinics to the Eugenics Society—anything rather than to the hated British FPA. The Eugenics Society established the Marie Stopes Foundation and consulted Margaret Pyke as to the best use of the Whitfield Street premises. She served on the board for several years, a generous action considering the undisguised animosity Marie had shown her as Chairman of the FPA. The clinic became part of the Marie Stopes Memorial Centre where overseas nurses and midwives were taught. Three rooms were modified and equipped and courses were arranged in conjunction with the IPPF Europe Region on various aspects involving the health of women, marital problems, venereal disease and, of course, contraception. Helena was responsible for the courses on contraception, and also did one session a week in the birth control clinic.

The courses were held every other month and comprised an introductory three-day period of technical instruction, followed by five days' practical training. Women were engaged as paid human models and Helena used her own plastic model. The project proved so successful that in addition to doctors from overseas, midwives already in the United Kingdom for training who would then return to their country of origin were also admitted on a quota. Helena would give a preliminary introductory training session and the students would then attend a number of practical sessions at the London hospitals where the European Region of the IPPF was responsible for family planning clinics. Helena set the standard for selection of students and agreed the quota. Many midwives were unaccustomed to examining women who were not pregnant and the foreign midwifery students had also to learn more than nurses in the United Kingdom because on their return home they would have greater responsibility in remote rural conditions, where they might have only infrequent contact with a doctor. They therefore had to be trained to fit intra-uterine devices and to prescribe the contraceptive Pill.

In 1960 Mrs Joan Windley, who had been Marie Stopes's secretary for most of her professional life, was appointed Administrator of the clinic, later to become Director responsible for the day-to-day running of the clinic and the various activities carried out including training at the Marie Stopes Memorial Centre. She had known Helena previously and remembered her with affection:

She was amazing but not easy to work with because she had her set views though she was much less opinionated than Marie Stopes. These people who achieved so much were eccentric. They had to be to do what they did. Whenever I asked for help, Helena gave it me, not by taking any action herself, but by encouraging me to talk over a particular problem. She used in those days to arrange third party adoptions. When I asked her advice about arranging a third-party adoption (hoping she would take it on herself) Helena's reply was that as a responsible member of the public I should see it through myself, calling on her for help if needed.

Personal communication to the author—1.6.82

The Royal College of Nursing was later to show interest in training nurses in the field of contraception and, according to Mrs Windley, Helena encouraged this at the Memorial Centre, somewhat unexpectedly in view of her early battles with Marie Stopes. However, by the time Marie died Helena had evidently become converted to Marie's theory that nurses could relate to women better than doctors could. Mrs Frances Solano, the outstanding chief nurse who worked with Helena at the Stopes Memorial Centre, loved Helena and in turn was greatly respected by Helena, although as Mrs Solano told me:

Dr Wright was not lovable in the conventional sense; she was too strict and autocratic, but the models and the girls loved her and enjoyed her sense of humour, just as I did. She commanded great respect and was a marvellous teacher, very hard working, not interested in fees although it was a private clinic. She had great empathy with the coloured girls, including many Africans, on the courses.

Personal communication to the author—1.6.82

According to Mrs Solano, Helena established less accord with some overseas male doctors whom she found arrogant: they got short shrift if they gave themselves airs. A Bulgarian doctor got his hand slapped by Helena, who thought he was examining a patient roughly. 'I professor,' he growled. 'She not do that.' 'Just sit over there and keep quiet,' was all Helena said, as reported by Mrs Solano.

I could believe Helena when she repeatedly told me she preferred women to men, but I was not convinced that she was as prejudiced against the male sex as she sometimes chose to appear. However, the

229

paediatrician (now Professor) Roy Meadow of Leeds University made me wonder if this attitude may have been more than a superficial pose. On an FPA course in 1962 he found himself the only man among twenty-nine young women doctors sitting at Helena's feet.

She was introduced by the tutor rather as a guest artist—'The Grande Dame of Contraception'. My mind went back to the days when I was in the cadet force at school and Montgomery came along to talk to us at a CCF camp. We were expected to bow as if we knew all about Alamein. The lecture proceeded and Helena Wright told us that women did not only come to clinics for advice about birth control. They came to the family planning experts as to 'mother figures', as they saw them. Suddenly Helena Wright saw me, caught my eye, and it was clear that she had not considered a family planner as a 'father figure' in any sense, and that if she had, she did not fancy the idea.

One went to various clinics on this course and I met her again. I had just finished two years of house jobs at Guy's and was very used to examining women. I had just got my diploma in obstetrics, but she treated me as if I was a medical student . . . You know how arrogant you are as a houseman, but I was not sure if she was so patronising because I was a man, or because a lot of women had been out of medicine for a while and were rusty, so she thought she had to start at the bottom. Anyway she wasn't in tune with my particular level. I don't know if the women thought this, but I do know they liked her. She was a very likeable lady.

Once she lifted up her plastic model and a lot of Dutch caps popped out of the trap door and bounced about all over the room. I can remember her exclaiming, 'Oh dear, they *are* active today!'

The course was very useful though and, although womanly aspects were overstressed, in my day medical students got no information about family planning at Guy's, and even in my six months as an obstetric and gynaecological house surgeon, there was no talk whatsoever about birth control.

Personal communication to the author—2.7.81

By the Sixties the newer methods of contraception, the Pill and the intra-uterine device, were being widely used. Not that the IUD was a new method: the Egyptians had known about it for over two thousand years and used to insert small stones into the uteri of camels, so that they would not become pregnant and therefore lazy during the long desert treks. But the Pill was certainly an innovation which revolutionised the whole practice of contraception.

In the latter part of the Fifties the Catholic Boston obstetrician Dr John Rock, and the physiologist Gregory Pincus, working in laboratories in Worcester, Massachusetts, established the effectiveness of the synthetic ovarian hormones, oestrogen and progesterone, given by mouth at regular intervals, in temporarily suppressing ovulation by the same biochemical action which naturally stops the release of eggs in pregnancy. Pincus's work on rabbits and rats was followed by large-scale clinical trials in Puerto Rico as a result of which the Pill came into general use in 1956 in the USA. In 1958 Pincus delivered the first major lecture on oral contraception in the United Kingdom. After further trials by the Council for Investigation of Fertility Control of the FPA, of which Dr Beric Wright was the Secretary of the Technical Sub-Committee, the Pill became available in 1961. This marked the turning-point in the medical opposition to contraception by those doctors who had never liked the cap and now found they had only to write a prescription.

In England Dr Margaret Jackson had been responsible for much of the early evaluation of the Pill and spoke on the subject in 1964 at a regional conference of the IPPF in London. It was estimated that four million people had taken the Pill since the first trials in Puerto Rico ten years previously. Margaret Jackson's comparison in 1964 of the effectiveness of contraceptive methods in use put the Pill at the top of the list, closely followed by the IUD; then came the condom, only slightly more effective than the diaphragm, which was not considered in this survey much better than *coitus interruptus* although in greater favour with the family planners, especially Helena, who thought the diaphragm preferable to the IUD. Foams and vaginal spermicides came low on the list, with the rhythm method at the bottom.

According to Mrs Solano, Helena did not fit the intra-uterine device but she did prescribe oral contraceptives. She was meticulous in applying safeguards in using the Pill in the light of the current knowledge—or lack of knowledge—of its possible dangers. In the early Sixties reports of side effects were reaching the public through the press, particularly in America. Contrary to certain medical advice Helena's successor on the IPPF Central Medical Committee urged the IPPF to put out a prematurely sanguine statement of reassurance. It is questionable if Helena would have supported this. She amplified her reservation about the Pill when speaking to an Indian Medical audience in 1977:

> The Pill [was] the first 100 per cent reliable contraceptive. As such it was an enormous advance. But because it was 100 per cent effective it altered the whole of society. It was responsible for the sexual revolution in the West and has become the foundation stone of the permissive society, as such to some people almost holy and above criticism. Over the years bit by bit we have discovered side effects of the Pill. They as you know are numerous and sometimes very serious . . . But how terribly difficult it has been to get these side effects known to doctors, let alone the public . . . I object strongly to those who have in my opinion whitewashed it, and continue to press for it to be available without a doctor's prescription on the grounds that it is quite harmless . . . I think the Pill is valuable in spacing children, real family planning, but taken as it is in the West it cannot be good . . . I totally support Family Planning but bitterly oppose the situation in England where women are not told the truth about the Pill; in fact there appears to be a deliberate suppression of the full facts—almost a conspiracy of silence.

For Helena barrier methods, combined with a chemical spermicide, remained her method of choice. Here again she set the pattern of later informed opinion, for by the Seventies the cap and condom had been raised to favour in view of doubts about the Pill and the IUD.

Although Helena attended all the IPPF international and regional conferences, she seldom presented a formal paper. Her contributions were largely confined to informal discussions and to teaching. However, in 1966, fifteen years after she had given her major paper in Bombay, she returned to the platform at a regional conference in Copenhagen. This time she included male contraception and laid out her rules for the use of the condom to her medical audience.

> If a sheath is to give complete protection against pregnancy, the following points must be observed on every occasion:
> (1) The sheath must be put on the erect penis before there has been any contact whatever between the tip of the glans penis (which potentially can harbour a number of sperms) and the moist parts of the vulva.

(2) At the first movement of penetration the man must hold the rim of the sheath and make sure that it stays in place during insertion into the vagina.

(3) Withdrawal from the vagina must take place before the penis becomes limp otherwise the sheath inevitably slips off into the vagina, and maximum danger is incurred by the escape of semen from the empty sheath.

(4) When withdrawal has been safely accomplished, the sheath must be removed, and the penis most carefully and thoroughly dried before it is safe for the two to lie together face to face.

Of these indispensable rules, the two most commonly broken are the first and the third. It should therefore be obvious that a chemical spermicide should habitually be inserted into the vagina before intercourse begins.[10]

The following year Helena returned to this theme at an IPPF International Conference in Santiago, giving the same instructions on the use of the condom as before. A medical audience would surely have understood the basic finger and glove principle involved, but her fourth rule is hardly realistic. Most surprisingly of all, no mention was made of the paramount importance of holding on to the rim of the condom during withdrawal from the vagina, as is now universally accepted and advised by the manufacturers in their printed instructions given with the product. One likely explanation for Helena's omission of this basic provision is that she had no personal experience of condom-protected intercourse. While she relied on her sexual partners for emotional and intellectual support, it would have been out of character for her to expect, let alone allow, them to take contraceptive responsibility.

While Helena was working at the Marie Stopes Clinic, not only was she particularly interested in the quality control of spermicides for use with caps and condoms but, according to Mrs Solano, she continued to press the manufacturers to insert instructions in condom packs. A British Standards Institution Technical Committee on Contraceptives was set up in 1959 and reported in 1964 without making any stipulations regarding instructions for the use of condoms. It was not until 1972 that the British Standards Institution main revision of the

[10] Helena Wright. Proceedings, Fifth Conference of Europe and Near East Region of the IPPF, Copenhagen, 5–8 July 1966.

'Specification for Rubber Condoms' repaired this omission. However, by the late Sixties the condom manufacturers, London Rubber Industries, had already begun to put instructions in with their packs. It is not unduly fanciful to trace Helena's influence here. In 1982 Mr Ian Locke who joined the London Rubber Industries in 1968 could still recall amusing conversations with Dr Helena Wright.

While actively engaged in furthering the world movement and as Vice-President of the IPPF, Helena had also found time to write her last book, *Sex and Society*. It had taken her four years. She asked Sir Theodore Fox, former Editor of the *Lancet*, to write the foreword. To Helena's chagrin he declined, being unwilling as its Director for the FPA to appear to support such a controversial book, and it was published in 1968 without a foreword. While it was still in typescript Sir Theodore had mentioned the book in his closing address at the Copenhagen Regional IPPF Conference, when he referred to Helena as 'no less a pioneer today than thirty years ago'. His theme was 'Educating the Educators', and he asked:

> Has the time come, in fact, when we should radically revise all our ideas of sexual relationships in the light of what one may call the contraceptive revolution? . . . Some of you may have doubts about any general tolerance of premarital intercourse. Some of you, though grateful to Dr Wright for pointing to the eventual consequences of contraception, may feel that the new type of marriage she foretells is something not for tomorrow, but at earliest the day after.[11]

Sir Theodore was not alone in questioning Helena's assumption that because she was free of possessiveness and jealousy, others could accept extra-marital relationships with equanimity, although in fairness it must be remembered that she laid down certain important reservations in her 'new code'.

Being Helena she accepted Sir Theodore's refusal philosophically:

> Dear Sir Theodore,
> After recovering from the first disappointment and reading your letter several times, I found that I agree with your opinion about a foreword. It is a relief to know that I will not be involving anyone else in whatever reactions the book may inspire in

[11] T. F. Fox. Proceedings, Fifth Conference of Europe and Near East Region of the IPPF, Copenhagen, 5–8 July 1966.

unpleasant directions. You are right, I much prefer to be solely
responsible . . .

HRW to T. F. Fox—27.11.67

Her letter went on to criticise 'the orthodox opinions and lack of
imagination' of the students at University College Hospital where, on
Sir Theodore's instigation, she had recently given a lecture on contraception at a Student Christian Movement meeting. She had told her
'Christian' audience that uncontrolled maternity was 'a fatal disease'
that affected the wife, the children, and ultimately the world. She
cited the world population figure of 3,000 million which unless
'controlled' would double itself in fifty years, saying that 100 million
births were expected in the current year and that for every death two
children would be born. She postulated that 'population control is
essential for the future of the world'—evidence of some change of
heart from earlier pronouncements.

She was soon back to the need to separate sexual intercourse from
reproduction and developed her theme that 'Marital experience can
ultimately be ruined by fear of pregnancy, leading to alienation of
husband and wife, with gradual withdrawal of the wife from any
happy participation in sex activity.' Helena then elaborated her
concept of the reasons underlying the Roman Catholic attitude

> . . . [which] approaches a very deep, complicated part of human
> psychology and is concerned with the fatal tendency to connect
> pleasure with guilt, which has always been specially strong
> where sexual pleasure is in question. I suggest further that as all
> the opinions and dogmas and teachings of the Roman Catholic
> Church have been put together and are being taught by *men*, that
> as the vast majority of these men are priests, self-condemned to
> celibacy, it is hardly likely that such a body of people *could* have
> much understanding . . .

Sir Theodore Fox's next letter must have softened the blow of its
predecessor:

> Dear Dr Wright,
> I want to let you know how very grateful I feel for your letter.
> It's sad the UCH students were so orthodox . . . but the Sec-
> retary was unquestionably right in suggesting that you shook
> them.
> Both in forming (and unforming) opinion and in helping

patients you seem, if I may say so, to be using your gifts to great advantage.

Yours very sincerely

T. F. Fox to HRW—Green House, Rotherfield, Sussex, 3.12.67

So, would Sir Theodore have written her foreword if he had not been Director of the FPA at that time? Apparently not:

My only virtue as an editor is that I can see other people's points of view, and I saw hers. But if you ask me if it had my approval I think I must say 'no'.

Personal communication to the author—6.12.82

Throughout her life Helena never wavered in the face of obstacles or criticism, and the IPPF rewarded her. In 1973 it established three Founders Awards to mark its twenty-first anniversary. These awards were given in the names of those who had been most active in promoting different aspects of planned parenthood: Elise Ottesen-Jensen of Sweden, Dhavanthi Rama Rau of India and Helena Wright of Great Britain. Thus Helena took her rightful place among the giants. There were some IPPF activities Helena did not want to support, and during conversations with Mr Carl Wahren, the Secretary General, who came to visit her at her home on 22 April 1980, she asked for her award to be assigned to the bi-monthly information sheet, the IPPF *Medical Bulletin*, in order 'to secure the continued and expanded dissemination of contraceptive knowledge to doctors throughout the world'. In the year of her ninety-third birthday the IPPF made her Patron of the *Medical Bulletin*, and her name remained on the masthead until her death.

Later Interests

Helena's enlarging practice was not confined to the contraceptive field and included distressed girls who were pregnant, and women who wanted to become pregnant but failed to do so. A number of these pregnant girls asked for an abortion. Early in 1957 she began to bring together the two groups and to arrange for childless couples to adopt the unwanted babies. These 'third party' adoptions were provided for under the Adoption Act of 1958 and remained legal in spite of a strong campaign to outlaw them, until the Children Act of 1975 was implemented in 1982. They had long been unpopular with both the local authorities and the registered adoption agencies whose social workers bitterly resented what they considered to be meddling by amateurs, and in some instances even suspected the practice as constituting illegal 'baby farming'. In Helena's time some doctors were undoubtedly making money by arranging adoptions and so breaking the law. The abolition of third party adoption was the culmination of a century of legislation designed to prevent trafficking in children, which had once been a profitable industry.

Helena would certainly not admit to amateur status and in her role of third party considered she was acting professionally in the interests of her patients. The demand for babies exceeded the supply, but through other doctors, youth clinics and acquaintances, Helena got to hear of a number of pregnant single girls who were only too glad to learn of someone prepared to adopt their babies when they were born. Whereas today the single mother is accepted in society, helped and encouraged to keep her child, the stigma carried by illegitimacy was still strong in the Sixties. Out of kindness the Wrights gave several single girls shelter during the war and employed them at 5 Randolph Crescent as domestics. Helena would fix the girl's admission to a maternity hospital and arrange for the baby to be adopted. She tried to place the baby as soon as possible, before the mother became attached to her child, and, if she could have bypassed the regulations, would have liked to do this on the first day after birth instead of leaving the baby in the maternity home or hospital, or in a mother-and-baby home.

Her routine practice was to interview the childless couple at some length, enquire into their medical history and ensure that they had a good reason for wanting to adopt a baby. She would then put the couple on a waiting list until a baby turned up for adoption. She insisted that all adoptive parents should instruct solicitors to carry out the legal obligations of the Adoption Act, and left it to the local authorities to inspect the homes of the adopters. When the time came to hand over the baby the mother would bring or send the baby an hour before the adopters were expected, and leave without seeing them. Helena's secretary would then transfer the baby to the adoptive parents. Helena's policy was to place the child as soon as the hospital considered it ready to be discharged. Her own responsibility ended when the Court Order for adoption was completed, but she would keep 'in friendly touch' if the parents wished.

Until the Abortion Act of 1967 and the effect of the Pill virtually eliminated the supply of babies, Helena completed some thirty-five third party adoptions. All the babies were illegitimate, except in one case where the mother already had four children and could not afford to bring up a fifth. The other girls were unmarried, apart from one who had a brutal husband and whose lover repudiated the child. Helena had met the girls in the early stages of pregnancy when they were seeking an abortion as the only alternative to adoption. There was no possibility in their circumstances of keeping the baby and where it was possible Helena would confirm this with the girl's mother, making sure the potential grandmother realised she was rejecting the unborn child.

Among the girls for whom Helena arranged a third party adoption was one called Geraldine who had been living and working at Randolph Crescent. Three days after the birth Geraldine wrote from the hospital saying that when the baby was ten days old she could 'come home':

Dear All,
. . . Patricia is fine and so am I . . . I'm glad Dr Wright is pleased and hope she will come soon to see her. She will like her . . . Mr Wright came on Sunday, but could not stay long enough

for me to thank him for bringing me to hospital and for the lovely box of chocolates.

I'm sure the lady will like Patricia as she is cute and very quiet . . . Please come and see her one day. She is lying in her cot and grinning at me and ready for another bottle.

Love to everyone at No. 5

From Geraldine and Patricia

3.12.60

The Obstetric Registrar at the hospital had already informed Helena of the birth of Geraldine's baby and confirmed that lactation was being suppressed, as arranged. He reported that he had unfortunately had to comply with the mother's 'emphatic insistence' on bottle feeding the baby herself. He had notified the adopters and suggested they should telephone on the eighth day.

Helena was evidently not familiar with, or turned a blind eye to, the provision of the 1958 Adoption Act which under Section 40 required anyone who wished to place or receive a child for adoption to give fourteen days' notice in writing of the intention to do so to the local authority, except in emergency when notice had to be given within seven days after placing the child with the adopters. The statutory fourteen days' notice allowed the social workers to investigate the suitability of the adopters and enabled the authority to forbid the adoption in the interests of the child if conditions were found to be 'detrimental'.

Helena ran into trouble when she failed to give the London County Council fourteen days' notice before she placed Geraldine's baby with her chosen adopters. The omission was noted when, *after* receiving Patricia, the prospective adopters duly notified their intention to apply for an adoption order. 'I do not propose to take any further action,' wrote the L C C Area Children's Officer to Helena on 4 January 1961, 'but I should like your assurance that the statutory notice will be given in any future placing.' Helena apologised, accepted responsibility for her negligence and undertook not to let it happen again. 'Unfortunately I don't seem to have been informed by anyone who the local authority concerned was,' she wrote plaintively, 'perhaps you would let me know how to find out before the next child is born.' On another occasion when Helena omitted to give the fourteen days' notice, the adopters had telephoned the London Borough of Redbridge, advising the authority that they would be receiving a baby

239

from Helena in four days' time. The Redbridge Children's Officer acted swiftly and sent Helena an extract from the Adoption Act 1958 including Section 40, and detailing also Section 44 which sets out the penalties for infringement. He enclosed a form for her completion and expected 'to be informed that the placing of this child is to be delayed in accordance with the law'.

Helena's knowledge of the Adoption Act may have been rudimentary but she was quick to discover the loophole in the escape clause which covered an emergency situation. Not surprisingly, her definition of an emergency differed from that of the social workers. She was, of course, motivated only by her desire to get the child placed as soon as possible and was prepared to rely entirely on her own judgement. The Croydon Children's Officer made clear his views when Helena told him she regarded the simultaneous discharge on the same day of a mother and baby from a maternity home, when the home refused to keep the baby, as an 'emergency'. 'Although I do not wish to prohibit you from placing this child,' he wrote on 13 February 1967, 'this is not to say that I regard the circumstances you have described as an emergency and I propose to seek further advice on this question.' The following year, when Helena notified the same official (within the statutory period) of her intention to place another baby, he sent her a lengthy interpretation of the working of the Adoption Act and her obligations thereunder. By then she must have become a byword among the professional social workers involved in adoptions.

She had fought one of her early battles with Miss Amicia Carroll, the Hampshire County Children's Officer. Miss Carroll discovered at the end of 1962 through one of her child care officers who had been called to see a lady in Milford-on-Sea, that this lady's name was on Helena's waiting list for a baby. Miss Carroll disapproved and wrote to Helena to say so on 7 December 1962:

> The experience of my staff is that several adoption societies are making placements in the county, and that childless couples able to offer a happy and secure home do not seem to be meeting difficulty or undue delay in their applications. In these circumstances there does seem to be reason to think that couples who look elsewhere for children to adopt are very likely to be those whose emotional or other problems would be revealed by the kind of enquiry an adoption society or local authority would make.

Miss Carroll did not feel able 'at the present time' to advise for or against an adoption arrangement for the couple concerned, but she felt bound to draw Helena's attention to 'the grave risks' to children placed in the care of couples seeking in the child 'a means of alleviating their own emotional (and possibly matrimonial) problems'. The crux of the matter turned out to be that a child placed by Helena had recently been committed to the care of the Hampshire Authority 'in circumstances which could have had more than disastrous consequences for the child and only slightly less for the adoptive mother'. It was clear to Miss Carroll that the enquiries before placement had not been 'as thorough as possible' in the previous adoption.

Helena was enraged and immediately demanded to know to whom the County Children's Officer was referring. All Miss Carroll would say was that she was not at liberty to reveal her name, but that the adoptive mother had suffered 'a severe mental breakdown involving great danger to the child', and had received treatment in a mental hospital. In the circumstances she could not recommend her authority at that stage to place a child with the lady in Milford-on-Sea who was on Helena's waiting list. She suggested that it might be better to know the couple better before reaching a decision. Finally Miss Carroll thought that perhaps help from a Family Planning Clinic might enable them to have a natural child, 'which I am sure you will agree would be the most desirable thing that could happen'.

Helena immediately wrote to the County Medical Officer of Health, demanding to know 'by what right, custom, or authority, is a Children's Officer allowed to withhold important information about a private patient of a doctor':

> As I have for five or six years been concerned with a number of adoption cases, all of which have turned out brilliantly successful, I am naturally extremely disturbed at not being allowed to know what has happened to the only one of my patients who is said to have had any trouble.

> HRW—7.1.63

There is no evidence that Helena ever discovered the identity of her patient, but she did succeed in providing the couple from Milford-on-Sea with a baby after all. Sixteen months later, on 16 May 1964, Helena's secretary, Joyce Whittle, handed a baby together with his birth certificate over to them for adoption.

In February 1962 Helena ran doubly foul of the law when she failed, once more, to give the statutory fourteen days' notice, or indeed any notice at all, to the Oxfordshire County Council in respect of a proposed adoption. The Children's Officer learnt only from the prospective adopters that Helena was about to provide them with a baby and that the baby was to be one day old. While complaining to Helena about her failure to notify her, the Children's Officer hoped that a child would not be placed until due notification had been received and drew attention, as others had done, to Sections 40 (1) and (3) of the Act. She added that she was 'somewhat concerned' to learn that the baby was to be only a day old as she would not have thought that 'one-day placing was the right time either for the mother or the baby'.

The Children's Officer then discovered, when calling on the proposed adopters, that Helena had charged them five guineas, thus violating Section 50 of the Act which expressly forbade payment in any form by either party. As a result the Oxfordshire Children's Officer informed the adopters' solicitors that if the proposed adoption were to go forward, she would have to report the payment of the fee to the court. The solicitors conveyed this information to Helena:

> . . . It follows from this that there is a possibility (I cannot of course put it higher than this) that the Court might direct that either you or my clients should be prosecuted under Section 50 of the Act . . . My clients naturally feel that they would not want to run the risk (however slight it might be) that they might be prosecuted . . . and with the greatest regret decided that they cannot proceed with the adoption . . .
>
> Once again may I say that the whole position has caused them great concern and disappointment.

Mortally offended, Helena again pleaded ignorance to the Children's Officer:

> . . . In the five or more years that I have been successfully conducting adoptions, no one has mentioned the Section 50 of the Adoption Act; on the contrary all the solicitors, magistrates and children's officers concerned have been completely satisfied that all the procedures were legal and in perfect order.
>
> I am in private practice as a gynaecologist. People write for appointments from all over England and many other countries . . . Mr and Mrs M. wrote to me asking if I would see them and

give my opinion as to whether I thought they were fitted to be adopting parents . . . I gave them a consultation of about an hour . . . and then gave . . . my opinion that they were suitable adopting parents. From my point of view this consultation was an ordinary professional occasion and the fee of five guineas is the usual one for such a consultation. As I have no idea as to what are the provisions of Section 50 I cannot guess in what sort of way I am considered to have disobeyed them . . .

Helena Wright, MRCS, LRCP, MB, BS (Lond.)

6 p.m., 21 February 1962

Eight years later financial queries were raised again when the Children's Officer of the London Borough of Tower Hamlets was involved in another adoption. On 13 January 1970 she wrote to Helena to thank her for the notification though she was a 'little concerned' that it came after the baby had been with the adopters for four days. She was also 'rather confused about the money involved'. Would Helena kindly let her know 'a little of the background details . . . as our report will have to be submitted to the Court'. As a result Helena sent back to the proposed adopters a cheque for seven guineas, explaining to them that when she had seen them for the first and only time two years previously and charged them this sum, she was considering them as private patients. 'Later I was informed by authorities in connection with the Adoption Act that fees are not payable even to a doctor if the purpose of the visit is to ask for and make preliminary arrangements about an adoption.'

Helena's actions in another case came to the attention of the Director of Public Prosecutions, and she was interviewed by Detective Sergeant John Pole from New Scotland Yard on 6 January 1968. Helena made a long statement in which she admitted that a prospective adopter and a single girl had each paid her small sums in consultations. Helena explained that over the past ten or eleven years she had seen many couples who would like to adopt children, and pregnant unmarried girls. They were accepted as private patients and paid the appropriate fee of seven guineas (fellow practitioners and medical students free; doctors' wives and nurses half fees).

The case under police investigation differed from others she had handled only in that the baby had already been born, and that a stranger who had heard of Helena through her work at the Marie Stopes Memorial Centre introduced to her the mother and the prospective adopting couple. She, Helena, understood that the un-married girl came in order that Helena might be able to find suitable parents to adopt her child. At the same visit Helena instructed the girl in an appropriate contraceptive method and proposed to see her in future once a year. The girl agreed to be a private patient and paid the seven guineas. The following day the couple involved came to see Helena and were judged to be suitable adopters. As private patients they too paid the seven-guinea fee, and Helena gave them a letter to the Children's Officer at Richmond. Her statement concluded:

> In the organisation of these adoptions, which often take months and involved much correspondence and telephone calls, there are inevitable expenses which I pay personally. Therefore I feel that when these persons come to me for help, which very often entails my talking to them for at least an hour, it is only right that they should pay me the usual consultation fee for my time. These people are astonished to hear that all the necessary negotiations are done for them free with no other expense other than the original consultation fee.
>
> I should like to say that if I have, with all good will, inadver-tently done anything that I ought not to have done, I offer my sincere apologies.
>
> H. R. Wright, 16 January 1968

In due course Helena was prosecuted under Section 50 of the Adop-tion Act. She had technically broken the law, albeit for a very small sum, but was not prepared to recognise that by taking what she regarded as a normal consultation fee, she was arranging an adoption 'for reward'.

She was defended by the Medical Defence Union and represented by Mr James Comyn, QC (later a High Court Judge), the MDU having decided that a doctor of Helena's distinction deserved lawyers of equal distinction. Helena, who took a somewhat arbitrary and quixotic view of the Adoption Law, proposed, against their legal advice, to plead not guilty when the case was heard at Wells Street Magistrates' Court on 2 April 1968. The solicitor acting for the MDU, Mr Peter Baylis, remembered Helena arriving in a cantankerous mood. Why, she wanted to know, should she plead guilty to breaking a law of which she disapproved? If the Law was an ass the lawyers probably were asses too. Mr Comyn eventually managed to persuade her at the very door of the court to change her mind, and she did plead guilty to one charge. Mr Comyn explained to the court that his client was a distinguished gynaecologist who was not engaged in improper adoptions, and gave an assurance that she would not charge consultation fees in any future adoption arrangements. Helena received an absolute discharge in respect to one charge and no action was taken in respect to the others.

In 1973 two reporters from the *News of the World* posing as prospective adopters telephoned for an appointment. Peter Wright answered the telephone and, without consulting Helena, gave them one for 2.30 p.m. on 20 November 1973. When Helena tried to cancel it because she was no longer prepared to manage adoptions, she found her husband had written down the wrong address. Michael Litchfield and Sue Kentish duly turned up to discuss adoption and Helena felt she could not turn them away without at least hearing what they had to say. In any case she claimed she had no idea they came from the *News of the World*, although she had received a telephone message from the paper.

The story was published on 2 December 1973 under banner headlines:

The Scandal that will Shock Britain
WE SHOP FOR BABIES IN HARLEY STREET

The reporters were said to have interviewed a gynaecologist who had 'film stars, actresses and pop singers among his patients', and also Dr Helena Wright:

> She is a pioneer of the birth control movement. She is also a rebel. For Dr Wright . . . is an agent for private adoptions, short circuits normal procedure and hoodwinks the law. She even sets up a cloak and dagger handover operation of babies at her home . . . 'I know the adoption law backwards,' she told us, 'and I won't obey it . . . the law says there must be six weeks between the birth and the adopting parents taking away the baby, except in an emergency. I make them all emergencies and take the responsibility. You'd like a baby as soon as possible. Now working through my emergency business you can have the child on the third day. That's through me, not through anyone else. What we do is have the baby handed over in my house . . .'

The *News of the World* reported—correctly—that Helena disapproved of the way girls were kept with their babies in mother-and-baby homes for six weeks and had, said the reporters, outlined for them a way of infiltrating a home, finding an unhappy girl and asking her out to tea.

> 'That's your opportunity. You've got her out of the trap. Are you well off, or middling off or what? Have the mother and baby in your home and don't say what you think. Don't say anything about adoption yet. Now if all goes well, come back to me with the girl and I do the whole of the legal side.'

Helena was, of course, incensed. But even with the advice of the Medical Defence Union, and threatening the *News of the World* with the hypothetical power of the General Medical Council 'should it wish to take action', she got no reply to her protests to the editor, Peter Stephens, other than a brief acknowledgement of her letter. Mr Stephens merely wrote on 22 February 1974 that he was 'inquiring into the matters you raise'. The 'matters' were that the report was untrue and might be considered professionally damaging; Helena told Mr Stephens that she had written refusing to see 'Mr and Mrs Litchfield' but her letter had been returned as 'wrongly addressed'. 'As they had forced themselves in to my consulting room to discuss the Adoption Act I felt it would be bad manners to turn them out! The conversation began with my refusal to accept them as adoptive parents and I made no record of their visit.'

What had not come out in this report was that Helena arranged only one adoption after 1968, as her secretary Mrs Joan Leslie has testified. Although Mr Leo Abse, strongly supported by the National Children's Adoption Association, was busy sponsoring his private member's bill to outlaw private adoptions, the demand for homes had decreased since the passage of the Abortion Act of 1967, after which the supply of babies dwindled.

Instead of looking for adopters Helena was by then arranging some ten legal abortions a week. Joan Leslie's paperwork was increased by the need to notify these terminations on the statutory 'green card', but in fact the Abortion Act barely affected Helena's actions: it merely caught up with her established practice in that its provisions no longer required psychiatric endorsement. Faced with a desperate situation Helena was prepared to deal with it according to the dictates of her conscience. She was fearless where the law was concerned and welcomed the opportunity of saying what she thought in public, though she realised it could damage her reputation. She greatly admired Aleck Bourne for his much publicised abortion on the fourteen-year-old rape victim.

Her own activities regarding abortion had been the subject of a police enquiry as early as 1947 and are recorded in a statement made to Inspector G. Chestney and Detective Constable K. White of Central Office, New Scotland Yard on 23 December 1947. It concerned a Mrs A. S. for whom Helena had arranged for a gynaecologist to terminate the pregnancy. She had first seen the girl before her marriage in October 1943 and had fitted a contraceptive device, but Mrs A. S. did not return until March 1947, when she was pregnant for the fifth time. She had induced two miscarriages by injecting glycerine into the womb herself and on each occasion had had haemorrhages, necessitating emergency admissions to hospital. Helena consulted a fellow gynaecologist who agreed to terminate the pregnancy, which Helena justified on the grounds of Mrs A. S.'s past history and personality. As she told the police, she felt certain in her own mind that Mrs A. S. would undoubtedly attempt to procure another miscarriage: 'Mental strain . . . had so affected her psychological stability that . . . she was unable to stand the strain of a continued pregnancy and the likelihood of the birth and upkeep of a further child.' She did not need a psychiatrist to tell her that, she said. If the police officers were looking for someone out to make money they were disillusioned. Helena had charged Mrs A. S. four guineas in all, for five consultations.

Helena made no secret of her law-bending activities—or 'law-testing' as she called it—and was once heard to ask a colleague in ringing tones at a party, 'Who do you send your abortions to now X is in prison?' But in principle she was opposed to abortion, as she was to sterilisation which she looked on as a mutilation and evidence of the failure of contraception. As she told her Indian audience in 1977: 'It is quick and easy to scrape a live baby from its mother's womb, but it is much harder to scrape a dead baby from its mother's mind.'

There were, however, many instances before 1967 where abortion was the only solution if in her view the continuation of the pregnancy would ruin a girl's life. She established a team consisting of a psychiatrist and a surgeon who felt as she did, without any urge to profit financially—Helena was only prepared to deal with colleagues whose courage matched her own and who would stand by their opinions, as she herself did. It was her practice to give the girl a letter of introduction to the psychiatrist and wait for the report. If the pregnancy was to be terminated on psychiatric advice, she would then arrange this—if necessary finding the girl a cheap hotel for the night. Dr Jean Infield recalled that one evening when she called to see Helena at home, she found two unknown girls staying there who had had abortions earlier that day, and who had nowhere else to spend the night.

In 1961 Helena followed up one of her major interests, the problems of people serving prison sentences, by offering to give contraceptive advice to women in Holloway. The Governor, Mrs Joanna Kelley, and prison officials had for some time been aware that the prison service had lagged behind in not providing for women in prison the contraceptive services that were available in the general community. When hearing of the proposals a prison official complained that it would never do if the news got around that a gynaecologist in a women's prison was helping to make the work of prostitutes easier. Questions might be asked in Parliament. 'All the better,' replied Helena.

As usual, Helena made her own terms. A room was to be made available where she could see the girls entirely alone; they were to understand that she was nothing to do with the prison and that strict confidentiality would be observed. A room was fitted out in the basement and, as Mrs Kelley has remarked, 'Dr Wright thought it a tremendous joke to burrow down there on her own.'[1] Helena also greatly enjoyed the access this unpaid work gave her to girls whose babies were born in the prison maternity ward, where she was able to teach them how to avoid another pregnancy after their discharge from Holloway.

As a result of Helena's pioneering activities the Commissioners eventually revised the official policy and agreed that a prison doctor should provide contraceptive advice if requested. Before handing over her clinic Helena was able to teach the woman doctor appointed by the Home Office her methods and techniques.

In the early Fifties Helena had turned her attention to male prisoners in Wormwood Scrubs, believing with Arthur Koestler, who spent six weeks in Pentonville during the Fifth Column scare in 1940 and was also gaoled by Franco's supporters, that, 'The main problem is not fear of the hangman, it is the apathy, depression and gradual dehumanisation.' Helena conceived the idea of interesting prison

---

[1] Personal communication to the author—29.12.82

inmates in drama. Her friend Jon Haerem, whom she had introduced to Dr Joshua Bierer at the Marlborough Day Hospital in 1951, had produced a series of one-act plays which were acted there by out-patients who were undergoing psychotherapy. When Helena first knew Haerem he was an out-of-work actor who had become interested in directing plays. He was so successful in treating patients in this way that Helena, who had watched a performance, approached her friend, Dr John Mackwood, the psychiatrist at Wormwood Scrubs who had joined the staff at the prison originally at her instigation in 1943 when she found there were no psychiatric services there, and suggested that Haerem should be asked to help in the prison hospital. Dr Mackwood chose ten men who were undergoing group psychotherapy and Haerem brought along copies of a play he thought they might read aloud together. This proved to be a great success and no one wanted to stop at the end of the allotted time. The prison medical officer, Dr. J. Landers, sitting at the back, observed the animated response of one man serving a long sentence who had hardly spoken for two years. It was to be an exercise that was repeated many times.

In 1957 Jon Haerem, who by now was working in the prison education department and involved in the psychotherapy unit, put on *A Sleep of Prisoners* which was acted by prisoners in the hospital. The Governor, Gilbert Hair, who was watching with Helena, was so impressed that he asked for a second showing to which educationalists and Home Office representatives were invited. The following year Haerem produced *Waiting for Godot* in the prison hospital. Both plays had been chosen because they required an all-male cast.

The Governor eventually asked if Haerem would extend the project to men serving life sentences in the prison, and supported him when Haerem suggested that professional actresses might be invited to play the female parts. Accordingly Haerem put on *My Three Angels* and his friend Jane Aird volunteered to take the part she had played in the Lyric Theatre production, while three Scrubs lifers acted the convicts featured in the play. Other actresses have since helped, including Margaret Rutherford and Ethel Revnell. A mechanical stage has been built with dressing-rooms behind, and the plays have become an accepted part of the prison life. Jon Haerem received an MBE for his work at Wormwood Scrubs, which he attributed to Helena: 'I can't think what my life would have been without her and all the interesting things I have been able to do and the interesting people I have met through her. She was practical and warm, a wonderful, lovable person. Her indomitable spirit will be with me all my life. How fortunate I was to have known her.'[2]

Helena watched nearly every performance of the plays Jon Haerem produced, including the Wormwood Scrubs drama group's presentation on 24 June 1981 of its thirty-fourth production, *The Magic Cupboard*, a comedy in three acts by Percy Walsh. The audience consisted of some two hundred friends and relatives of prisoners and the cast included two professional actresses, Rosella Longinotti and Veronica Dimmock, while the male parts were played by men serving life sentences in the prison D-Wing. As the programme stated: 'The action takes place in the kitchen-parlour of a cockney family in Camden Town. The year is 1935 when one only needed a penny for a gas meter, 20 cigarettes cost one shilling (five pence today) and nobody owned a television set.' It took Helena back many years and it delighted her when, after the Governor's congratulations at the end of the performance, Jon Haerem rose to say, 'Nothing of this would have happened if twenty years ago Dr Helena Wright, sitting in the front row, had not introduced me to this work.' It was her last visit to Wormwood Scrubs.

In 1983 I made a pilgrimage to Wormwood Scrubs in Helena's path to see the Drama Group's presentation of their 37th production, *Off the Hook*. This farce, acted as usual by men serving life sentences, with professional actresses, deals with the antics of a pair of crooks who spring a man from prison. Their object is to find out from him where some stolen loot is hidden, but it fails when it transpires that they have picked the wrong man and the money had anyway already been handed over to the police. It was an amusing entertainment, and the cast whom I met had obviously enjoyed the performance as much as the audience. Helena's memory was still green and she would have appreciated the performers' pleasure. As the deputy governor said in his speech, 'Laughter is not often heard in prisons'.

---

[2] Personal communication to the author—29.12.82.

[13]
Last Years

When Helena was eighty-five she reduced her working days to three a week. Three years later, in 1975, the lease of her consulting room ran out, and she announced that she would not renew the ten-year lease the landlord offered. At the age of eighty-eight she had accumulated case notes of over 20,000 patients. These she deposited with the successor she had chosen twenty years before. She wrote to all her existing patients to tell them of her decision.

> This will be the last time that I will send you a letter of reminder. In December 1975 the lease of my rooms at 9 Weymouth Street expires, I will then be 88 and have decided to retire at the end of that month.
>
> Luckily for all of you, there will be no break in the availability of gynaecological consultations. Dr Jean Infield has promised me that she will take charge of any and all of my patients who wish for her advice and care. My association with Dr Infield is happy, confident and of long standing. In the early days of her medical experience she came to me at the Telford Road Clinic for teaching in contraceptive techniques. I quickly recognised her unusual ability and the sympathy and interest she shared in the human aspects of gynaecology. During the twenty years since that time, there have been many opportunities for her to demonstrate that my original estimate of her personality was justified. A number of my patients know her already, because she has often taken holiday oversight during my absences.
>
> Helena Wright
> October 1975

Helena's unpunctuality was the only criticism Mrs Leslie, who had known her as her secretary for five years, ever heard any patient make about her.

251

They were completely sold on her, and had complete faith in her, although many regarded her as eccentric. Helena was totally unshockable, but I sometimes wondered if the typical housewife would be equally unshockable when faced with Helena. What I most liked about working for her was her sense of the ridiculous, but she never caused offence and never lost her temper, though she could flatten with a few well-chosen words. I am terribly glad I knew her. I enjoyed her.

Personal communication to the author—2.12.82

Mrs Leslie worked for Helena during the Wrights' last years at Randolph Crescent. She used to arrive while the Wrights were having breakfast, to find a somewhat disorganised household run by one au pair girl who struggled inefficiently with, or else abandoned, the cleaning of the large house. Mrs Leslie, who had her desk in the dining-room, would go through the mail while Helena had her bath and then they did letters together for about an hour. Helena would leave her with the appointment book and the telephone, and would set off for her consulting room at least ten minutes after the first patient was due in Weymouth Street, driving like the wind in her characteristic single-minded style when set on any course in life. Mrs Leslie sometimes found her exacting in her tendency to use people. Helena had, for instance, discovered that dressmaking was Mrs Leslie's hobby and when work slackened off in the afternoons she persuaded Mrs Leslie to make clothes for her, which in fact she rather enjoyed. Mrs Leslie liked Peter but found him a 'rather pathetic old man. He was not working then and money was tighter.'

Mrs Leslie resigned in 1972. The Church Commissioners had not renewed the lease of Randolph Crescent and that year the Wrights moved to a small flat in Abbey Road in St John's Wood. It was in strong contrast to the spacious house in Randolph Crescent. There were three bedrooms and one living-room. Being on the ground floor it was convenient for Helena, who was beginning to experience pain from the degeneration of the cartilage in one knee. But she found their new living quarters cramped, particularly as she was still working, although less and less as time went on, and still needed space for her files and desk. She immediately christened the flat 'the Bird Cage'.

Helena replaced Mrs Leslie with Miss Mira Leslie, who was no relation, a gentle, artistic lady who came every morning to the Bird Cage, made the appointments from there for Helena's shortened working hours and typed her letters. She was the only person who refused to allow Helena to rechristen her. When she arrived Helena had told her in her usual fashion that she did not like the name Mira and would think up another one. 'No, thank you, Dr Wright,' was the response, 'Mira Leslie is my name,' and Miss Leslie she remained for the next ten years, becoming much more than just a secretary.

Peter had never been enamoured of the house in Randolph Crescent and spent relatively little time there latterly. He rather liked the Bird Cage. His practice had virtually evaporated before they left Randolph Crescent and he had retired from his hospitals although he went daily to his consulting room, perhaps to get away from Randolph Crescent. He had become melancholic in his later years, more so after an abdominal operation followed by complications the year before his death, and he was apt to be irritable. Miss Leslie described him as 'a dear, though rather irrascible'. When he accused her, as he sometimes did, of losing his things, Helena would tell her to look in his pockets, which was where the missing objects were often found. Helena, who had seldom cooked so much as an egg, now at eighty-five successfully cooked and cared for him with only daily help. She continued to go to Quainton at weekends and made arrangements for a particular friend to look after her husband.

On the afternoon of 10 August 1973 on her way to Quainton, Helena drove her Volkswagen through a red light at the junction of Western Avenue and Perivale Lane. This cost her her licence. She realised her error only when she heard her passenger, Daphne Charters who had lived on the top floor at Randolph Crescent, say quietly, 'The light is red.' Mrs Charters had psychic powers, and she and Helena were probably deep in conversation. Helena then turned obliquely right against the cross traffic and collided with three oncoming cars, one of which struck the nearside passenger door, breaking Mrs Charters's collar bone. Helena's left hand was bruised but no one else was hurt, although the car was a write-off. Two policemen took Helena and Mrs Charters to the Central Middlesex Hospital where, while Mrs Charters was being treated, the policemen took the opportunity of seeing if Helena could read a car number at twenty-five yards. She could barely manage twenty-three yards.

In view of what she described to the police as her 'unconscious failure of distant vision', Helena then promised never to drive again and there and then handed over her licence. The policemen got her a taxi and she and Mrs Charters drove on to Quainton. Since she had promised not to drive again Helena was annoyed to receive a summons to appear at Ealing Magistrates Court on 26 April 1974. She decided, however, to plead guilty, and wrote in reply to the Clerk to the Justices that, 'If the Justice of the Peace still thinks the case worth spending the Court's overworked time in hearing, I will be pleased to attend and to listen.' She was duly find £15 for 'driving without due care and attention' and £10 for 'failure to comply with an automatic traffic signal'.

Margaret Lowenfeld died on 2 February 1973. During much of her working life she had lived in London with her close companion and colleague, Miss Ville Andersen, who had originally come from Denmark as a student at the Institute of Psychology and had remained with Margaret Lowenfeld. On her mother's death Margaret had bought Cherry Orchards, a house at Cholesbury in Buckinghamshire which she used at weekends. As Margaret got older she and Ville Andersen spent more time there, and by 1970 she came to London to lecture only once a week. Her work diminished and she began to show evidence of deterioration, suffering increasingly from fantasies and alterations in mood. Two years before her death she had fallen out of bed, and Ville Andersen, who found her on the floor, heard her talking wildly in Polish about her school days, matriculation and Latin grammar. She remembered nothing of the incident but became progressively difficult thereafter.

It was clear to Helena that her sister was beyond recovery, and in 1972 she encouraged Margaret to move to a nursing home near the Wrights' flat. She spent Christmas that year with Helena and Peter in London and she died the following February, on the day before her eighty-third birthday in the Hospital of St John and St Elizabeth. She was in coma when her breathing stopped, but Helena who was with her remained convinced that she had been able to let her sister know that Bruce was 'waiting to accept her in a place of rest'.

Margaret Lowenfeld was buried in the graveyard of the church of St Lawrence at Cholesbury where Claire, the wife of her cousin Gunther Lowenfeld, is also buried. It is Lowenfeld country, near Gunther and Claire's home and near Little Brickhill where Margaret and Helena had spent the temporary release from Alice and Frank Quicke as schoolgirls; it is near their father's hunting lodge at Aston Abbots and it is fifteen miles from Quainton. Nine years later Helena was to lie in the same grave.

Their cousin, Ralph Beyer, the carver, who is known for his

architectural lettering in Coventry Cathedral, carved the inscription on both sisters' tombstones, as well as the commemorative plaque to Margaret Pyke at the FPA. Helena had learned in 1937 from Eric Gill that her young cousin, Ralph (the son of Margaretta, who was to die in Auschwitz) had come, a refugee from Nazi Germany, to Piggotts to learn carving and lettering as Gill's pupil. His parents could not help him from Germany, and when Beyer moved the following year on a very small grant to the Central School of Arts and Crafts (now the Central School of Art and Design), Helena gave him a home at Randolph Crescent. She later made him an allowance to cover his lodgings until he began working in the studio in Buckinghamshire of Donald Potter, another pupil of Gill's. Ralph Beyer was extremely grateful to Helena and, as he wrote after her death, 'It was she who enabled me to stay on in England and take up the work at which I was ultimately to make a living, and which has come to have some meaning in its own sphere . . . Her clarity of mind and complete candour . . . were always tempered by warm concern.'

Peter Wright died of bronchopneumonia on 3 May 1976. His death closed one of the several compartments in which Helena kept her life. His reputation may not have equalled Helena's but he too was distinguished in his own field and known internationally. He was a magistrate, a member of the Paris and Lyons Academies of Surgery, and Secretary for a long time of the British Association of Surgeons. He was influential in building up and was also Secretary of the International Society of Surgery. In 1945 de Gaulle made him a Chevalier de la Légion d'Honneur in recognition of his services to France and the French Hospital in London.

Helena always spoke of her husband with affection but without awareness as far as I could discover of the details of his achievements or beliefs. He undoubtedly came second to her career, as she had warned him he would at the time of their marriage. He had been raised among Plymouth Brethren and it cannot have been easy, and may have been impossible, for him to adjust to her unorthodox views, which must have affected their sexual relationship. A distinguished Swedish psychiatrist, Dr Thorsten Sjövall, who knew Helena well through the IPPF and at one time shared her views on sex, although he later changed his mind, believed that Helena's deep admiration and love for her father led her to accept his sexual behaviour and to think therefore that women had an equal right to disregard the conventions of society without considering the far-reaching consequences for the partner and the family. What Helena could or would not see was that others including her husband might not have the qualities this liberty demanded. It may indeed be that Peter would have been happier with a more single-minded and conventional wife, as his son Michael Wright has suggested, but a more forceful character might have offered objections to her life-style. As it was they were loyal friends who admired one another, and would never allow their marriage to break up.

Though she lived alone after Peter's death Helena was never lonely. She had numerous visitors and old friends and their children turned up at the Bird Cage from all over the world including India, America, Canada, China and Sweden. In spite of increasing pain in her knee which made her limp, and the onset of deafness, travel remained one of Helena's greatest pleasures in her later years. In 1971 she went to lecture in Beirut at the invitation of the gynaecologist, Dr Isam Nazer. Her contraceptive equipment was in her heaviest air-bag, and when Dr Nazer met her at the airport he told Helena it was illegal to bring these things into Lebanon, and if she wished to avoid them being confiscated next time she should bring the tools of her trade in her handbag! She did not meet many Lebanese but mainly members of organisations dealing with Palestinian refugee relief. The visit produced one unexpectedly good effect for Helena. Dr Nazer pointed out to her that if by using a stick she took the weight off her knee, which was now turning outwards, she could eliminate her pain, though not her lameness.

Even at the ripe old age of eighty-seven Helena was still travelling on behalf of the IPPF. Dr Ronald Kleinman remembered her energy when in 1974 she and Dr Margaret Jackson were guests of Dr Siva Chinnatamby, at the Twenty-first Anniversary Conference of the Sri Lanka FPA. Their plane arrived late but Helena, after a night in the air, went straight on arrival to the British High Commission for a lunch in honour of the British delegation. She made her seventh and last visit to India in 1978 alone when she was ninety, to visit her Calcutta friend Sita Chaudhuri, then up to Kalimpong, back to Calcutta and home to England in six weeks.

While she lived in the Bird Cage Helena continued as she had done for thirty years regularly, to visit Ceril Birabongse at Malcesine on Lake Garda. Her marriage to the racing driver Prince Bira of Thailand had been dissolved after twelve years and Italy had become her home. At the Villa Punta Campagnola Helena found peace and comfort in the loving company of Ceril 'who looked on me as a kind of aunt'. She used to spend the days painting, and from Princess Birabongse I learnt that Helena always had three paintings going at one time 'one for mornings, one for the afternoons and one for rainy days indoors'.[1]

Helena once described a typical day there in a letter to Bruce McFarlane who had twice come with her to Malcesine.

> . . . Yes—thank you—I'm having an ideal holiday . . . The eye meets nothing but delicate harmonies. Ceril's tiny maid Anna brings my breakfast tray at 8.30; the immense window (four panels) is fully open and I sit up or lie and watch the sun and the tree tops . . . I get up only when the wish comes. All the mornings I paint from the window at the north end. Lunch with Ceril in the garden, sleep and read and worship the mountains from my bed until about four. Come down and paint in the garden if not too hot, go walking along the old road, remembering you till dusk. Dinner indoors with Ceril and Bruno and immense discussions. We live in French. Bed when I like . . . There's so much beauty here that every minute is full . . .
>
> HRW to KBMcF—Punta Campagnola, 20.6.60

She would also visit her German family and friends or explore Europe with Adrian. When she was ninety-two she was able to fulfil a wish she had been hankering after since 1914 when the war prevented her joining her father in Bayreuth. She set off by herself to stay there with her cousin Rösel's son Till Haberfeld to hear his wife, the soprano Gwyneth Jones, sing Brunhilde in *Die Walküre* at the Festspielhaus. After the opera they sat up discussing the performance until 3 a.m. Gwyneth Jones was amazed at the originality and intelligence of the questions which Helena asked her.

> 'I want you to explain to me how you make a round tone, and how it is possible that the sound made by a choir boy, which is like a straight line, differs completely from that made by a dramatic soprano.' The intensity and precision of the question was very typical of Helena's permanent thirst for knowledge.
>
> Personal communication to the author—15.2.83

---

[1] Personal communication to the author—24.1.83.

Before returning to England Helena went on to Kronberg to see her god-daughter, Helena Harmsen, managing to command a wheelchair or a car at any airport where she needed them.

In 1977 Lady Medawar, Director of the Margaret Pyke Memorial Trust, arranged a party in honour of Helena's ninetieth birthday at the Margaret Pyke Centre in the FPA headquarters. Margaret Pyke, to whose inspiration the FPA owed its formation, had been its first Secretary and from 1954 to 1966 the Chairman of the National Executive Committee. She was succeeded at her death by Lady Medawar who, with Margaret Pyke's friends, raised the money for a memorial model training centre for study and training in family planning. The Margaret Pyke Centre, by then the largest family planning clinic in Britain, moved in 1980 into half the Soho Hospital for Women, a branch of the Middlesex Hospital. Helena duly attended the celebrations as an honoured guest with obvious enjoyment of her continuing recognition by her old FPA and IPPF colleagues and friends.

Later that year the Family Planning Association celebrated its Jubilee at a large reception at the Royal Society of Medicine in London. Helena was the only survivor of the six founding pioneers. Margaret Pyke was represented by her son Dr David Pyke, and Harry Stopes-Roe was also there. Margaret Jackson, though frail, had come from Exeter, and there were others who had worked with or been taught by Helena in the formative years. The Secretary of State, Patrick Jenkin, with many workers in the field of contraception, watched while Helena cut the celebratory cake amid acclamation —due recognition of her energy and vision fifty years ago, and marking the culmination of her early aspirations.

Helena had been interviewed that Jubilee morning on the BBC *Today* programme. She was an experienced broadcaster and the absence of 'well', 'oh' or 'er' confirmed the clarity of her mind. She spoke as flawlessly as many professional broadcasters. Four months later on 12 November, marking her ninety-third birthday, she was the guest speaker on BBC *Woman's Hour*. To the query as to whether 'at this splendid age' Helena felt her 'life's work' was finished, she replied somewhat predictably, 'Certainly not. We can say it's in mid career.' She told the interviewer that although to her sorrow she had had no daughter, luckily among her grandchildren there was one girl whose father and mother were both doctors.

Now last October she succeeded in becoming a medical student at my old hospital, the Royal Free. Now that worked out very neatly. It's exactly seventy years between the October this year and October 1910 when I also began in the same place.

In response to the interview many voices spoke from the past, among them Barbara Scott, now over eighty, who as the wife of a housemaster at Wellington College in the Thirties had suggested that her husband should invite Helena to speak informally on sex to the boys in his house—not incidentally with the entire approval of the Headmaster—and who had helped to persuade their friend George Turner, the Master of Marlborough College, to write the foreword to *What is Sex?* After the broadcast Mrs Scott wrote:

> Dearest Helena,
> You were splendid yesterday, the voice faintly different but the incisive statements just the same. You answered the questions with authority and spirit. I rejoiced and was proud . . . Congratulations on an impressive interview . . .

Others who wrote were a colleague, Dr Margaret Neal-Edwards who had not seen Helena since the IPPF Santiago Conference in 1967:

> I do congratulate you on your age and all your achievement. It has been a great joy to know you. We have lived through a wonderful century and you are one of the great ones in our profession . . . a woman in advance of your time. I am so glad you have lived to see the principles expressed in your books come into acceptance in Britain. It must have been a great source of satisfaction to you.

And Dr Colin Bertram, Dr 'Pip' Blacker's successor as General Secretary of the Eugenics Society, who first met Helena at the Bombay IPPF Conference in 1952:

> I am most certainly one of your admirers in all the good works you have done and leadership you have exerted over so many years . . . I only regret that Margaret Pyke was unable to achieve your splendid age and continued influence.

In speaking of her achievements in different fields, Helena omitted to tell the interviewer that she was already engaged in writing her seventh book, alas never completed. It was to be based on the social changes in the world over the previous fifty years, which demanded a wider approach than she had adopted in her early books. Now she intended to analyse the causes and effects of pornography, group sex, rape and other sexual crimes on society. We shall never know how this forward-looking ninety-three-year-old proposed to solve these and other problems except by education in sexual understanding.

In the same year, 1980, Helena went up to Birmingham by train to a meeting of the National Association of Family Planning Doctors. This organisation of which Helena and Dr Margaret Jackson were the first vice-presidents, was formed in 1975 to replace the medical council of the FPA when the clinics were taken over by the NHS. Dame Josephine Barnes who was also attending the Birmingham meeting remembered Helena 'sitting in the front row, smiling and obviously intrigued by the proceedings'. After the meeting, however, Helena proclaimed herself too tired to stay to the dinner which was to be held in the presence of the Mayor, and where a speech was to be made in which Helena would feature in some prominence. She was finally persuaded to change her mind by the promise that she would be taken to and from where they were staying in the Mayor's car, and in the event enjoyed herself so much that she stayed to the very end, returning at nearly midnight clutching an orchid.

In 1981 six members of a study group of four men and two women senior officials of the People's Republic of China Family Planning Association led by its Secretary General, Mr Wang Liancheng, arrived on a European tour. It was not until 1957 that Chou En-Lai had asked for birth control to be developed in China and the Chinese FPA had been in existence for only a year at the time of the London visit. Helena was invited to meet the party at a reception at the House of Commons on 11 May 1981, organised by the parliamentary group on population and development. She brushed up her Mandarin, rusty after fifty-four years, and put on a tidy frock. With their veneration for age, the Chinese were entranced by her. Helena also attended discussions on contraception the following day at the headquarters of the FPA where she was interested to learn that the Chinese in their drive for the one-child family were using the Filshie clip, which increases the chances of reversing the operation for sterilisation if required. Helena particularly admired the only member of the team who could speak English, the interpreter Miss Qiao Xinjian. To Mr Wang Liancheng Helena was able to say '*Ting hao*' (very good) and to Miss Qiao Xinjian '*Zaijian*' (goodbye), which greatly impressed them.

Helena spent her ninety-third birthday with Candida and Michael Wright at their Gloucestershire home. Candida had made five birthday cakes, one for nine-year-old Christopher Wright (14 September), one for her relative Eric de Maré, the photographer and writer (15 September), one for Adrian Wright (16 September), one for Helena (17 September) and Candida's own (18 September). Helena went to stay two or three times a year with this branch of her family who had offered to make a home for her if she became incapacitated, but although grateful she intended to die at Quainton which she looked on as her home. Unless she was going somewhere else she went to Quainton every weekend with Beric and his wife Sue, who would take her and fetch her back after she had ceased to drive her car. She relied increasingly on Beric at the end of her life and few days passed in London without a visit from him on his way to work. Adrian looked after her financial affairs and Beric her health and general welfare.

She spent the last Christmas of her life at Quainton. Michael and his family were there as well as Adrian. It was a happy time for her, a white Christmas, and everyone except Helena went for a walk in the sunshine. It was marred though by intimation of her approaching death in the shape of another of the feverish attacks which she had begun to experience, but she loved being with all her family. Daphne, who had been married to Christopher, came over to see her with the adopted children of her second marriage, and Helena was touched by their concern for her when she was not well enough to join them for lunch. On another day Margaret, Michael's first wife, came with Helena's granddaughter Miranda. On Boxing Day the Quainton bell-ringers rang carols in the big sitting-room, to everyone's enjoyment.

As Helena got older her appearance did not greatly change, but in her cousin Till Haberfeld's words:

> Her characteristics became more characteristic. Her mouth became thinner, the curious searching eyes more awake, the pointed masculine nose more dominant. Her personality still filled every room she entered. It was so strong her looks and clothes were unimportant by comparison. As Helena got older, I felt an increasing emotional warmth coming from her. I know few people who would sign a letter, as she did, 'Shining love! Helena' and I don't think she would have written to us in the same way ten years earlier.
>
> Personal communication to the author—15.2.83

At her advanced age her intellect was phenomenally sharp and she was still interested in every facet of life around her, children, friends, and their work. She never lost this facility and had even analysed the workings of a computer, leaving a diagram to illustrate this in her last year. She could still beat her gynaecologist grandson Jeremy at chess and she did not welcome telephone calls during a B B C chess programme. Her room in the Bird Cage was usually littered with books on subjects varying from travel, history, art and psychology, brought by the library visiting service, whose staff were magnetised by Helena's intellectual grasp of so many unrelated subjects. She sat up late at night because there was never enough time to read and would often telephone me around eleven p.m. She expected, and usually got, the best that life offered. She returned this in full measure.

There were many inconsistencies in her life, particularly her belief in paranormal manifestations and in life in the Fourth Dimension. It was difficult to make her illusions or delusions tally with the capable, practical scientifically-trained doctor that Helena undoubtedly was. Could she really believe, as she told me, that her friend Peggy Martland was using an electron miscroscope in 4D? When Helena used to describe her experiences with the paranormal, there always seemed to me a potential loophole to account for them. She left a carefully documented account of the disappearance on the day of a return from Quainton of a bottle of tablets she was taking from her bathroom in London, and its reappearance at Quainton the next weekend. Her conversation with Bruce McFarlane, then in 4D, convinced her that he had organised its dematerialisation in London and rematerialisation thirty miles away. Did she never think she might have had a temporary loss of memory and had left it all the time at Quainton? In 1977 while she was alone at Quainton she woke one night to find a fire had broken out on the ground floor. She went downstairs to telephone 999 and then discovered she had left her stick upstairs. She could not explain how she had managed the descent without it, unless Bruce and Peter had helped her. Yet the banisters at Quainton are made of strong wood and she only had to hold the rail for support.

Helena made several attempts to help people who were bereaved to get in touch with the departed, one of them being Princess Anne. Helena believed that animals could share an afterlife with human beings, as the following letter she wrote to the Princess when her horse Doublet was accidentally killed, indicates.

Madam,

To the numbers of letters of sympathy you will have had about the accident to Doublet I want to add one which perhaps will be a surprise.

Personal and individual survival after physical death is not limited to humans. Animals of any kind which have been able to develop sympathy and friendship with the people who care for them are also capable of surviving physical death.

You, therefore, have lost Doublet only in a physical sense. As far as I could judge from television and radio glimpses, you and Doublet have achieved real friendship. Nothing, of course, can lessen the sorrow and disappointment of having to live and to ride without his physical presence, but he himself, the unique personality who is Doublet, is alive and continually hoping for recognition from you. His physical world (a state with 4 dimensions instead of the three of ours) interpenetrates our world, and he (when he has recovered from the shock and surprise of his exit) will be often with you and probably always when you are riding. You may have discovered this piece of truth already by intuition. If so, I can confidently send sympathy and understanding. But if my statement is a surprise and difficult to believe, there is easy access in relevant libraries to many records, thoroughly well investigated, of incidents of communication between living people and their 'dead' animal friends.

I am your Royal Highness's humble servant.

HRW to the Princess Anne, Mrs Mark Phillips,
9 Weymouth Street, London 17.5.74

This letter was acknowledged with thanks on the Princess's behalf by her lady-in-waiting without further comment.

Helena had been in touch, as she claimed, with Bruce ever since she had caught his spirit immediately on finding him dead. After Peter's death she included him in their conversations, using the technique of 'telekinesis'. Holding a pencil loosely in her hand she would sit poised over a sheet of paper. 'Are you there, Bruce and Peter?' she would ask. According to Helena, when they were ready to speak her hand would move in such a way that she could not have moved it herself. She would then write down whatever they told her as long as their 'energy', which was apparently limited, sometimes only to fifteen minutes, lasted. The recorded conversations were uninformative about Bruce and Peter's actions on the other side in 4D, and appeared often to reflect Helena's own views or hopes. She had considered that the physical symptoms which arose in the year of her death might indicate she was about to join them. Not so, according to Bruce and Peter. They told her, wrongly, that she had first to finish her book and that she still had work to do on earth.

Helena had told her mother on Alice's sixtieth birthday that she, Helena, could 'with care and luck live to eighty, which is not much of an age'. She managed to exceed her own calculations by nearly fifteen years and on 23 March 1981 she died in the Royal Free Hospital after an operation for gall stones which was followed by complications. Miranda, working in the medical school for her second-year examinations, cheered her last days by her daily visits to her grandmother.

Helena was anxious to persuade someone on this side to promise to get in touch with her after death, as she and her mother had agreed to do. She believed the initiative should come from those on earth. She received limited encouragement from Michael and her much loved daughter-in-law, Candida. Michael did not believe, as Helena did, that this would be possible but, equally, he could not say that it was impossible and they agreed to do their best. Their efforts had not been crowned with success a year after her death, but Candida, who loved Helena deeply, was vividly aware of her presence during the evening on which she wrote this tribute for Helena's memorial gathering:

> Helena had a shining quality which was infectious: she and my great-uncle, Oliver Hill, were the only people I have known who seemed to have no regrets and no bitterness . . . They consciously applied themselves to what was before them in an individual way, because they were individual—undivided in the parts that made up themselves; and also undivided . . . from the people, places and events among which they were so alive.
>
> She delighted in things that were growing . . . personalities, plants and gardens, and new ideas at 94 . . . She did not resist the passing of time. Her convictions and motivations were entirely relevant to it . . . She lacked entirely the masculine driving forces of honour, pride and competitiveness . . . She had no great respect for men and their place in society but enjoyed their company. She respected most strength in women, and the independent self-possessiveness of cats, who can give

and take wholeheartedly on their own terms. Perhaps her most constant characteristic was the wholehearted attention to every companion and activity taken on, her feminine ability to listen and the masculine one to analyse what she had heard.

Bibliography

Brecher, E.M. and Brecher, R. *An Analysis of Human Sexual Response*. London, André Deutsch 1967.

Brecher, E. M. *The Sex Researchers*. London, André Deutsch 1970.

Ellis, Havelock. *Sexual Inversion (Studies in the Psychology of Sex)* Vol. 1 Watford Univ. Press 1897; Second Ed. Vol 2 Philadelphia, F. A. Davis 1901.

Ellis, Havelock. *Psychology of Sex*. London, Pan Books Ltd. 1967

Fryer, P. *The Birth Controllers*. London, Secker and Warburg 1965; London, Corgi 1967.

Gray, M. *Margaret Sanger: A Biography of the Champion of Birth Control*. New York, Marek 1979.

Griffith, F. *The Pioneer Spirit*. Upton Grey Green Leaves Press 1981.

Grosskurth, P. *Havelock Ellis: Stranger in the World*. London, Allen Lane 1980; Quartet Books 1981.

Hall, R. *Marie Stopes: A Biography*. London, André Deutsch 1977; Virago 1978.

Hall, R. (ed.) *Dear Dr Stopes: Sex in the 1920s*. London, André Deutsch 1978; Penguin Books 1981.

Kinsey, A. C., Pomeroy, W. B., and Martin, C. E. *Sexual Behaviour in the Human Male*. Philadelphia and London, W. B. Saunders Co. 1948.

Kinsey, A.C., Pomeroy, W. B., Martin, C. E., Gebhard, P.H. *Sexual Behaviour in the Human Female*. Philadelphia and London, W. B. Saunders Co. 1953.

Lambeth Conference 1930. Encyclical Letter from the Bishops with the Resolutions and Reports. Society for Promoting Christian Knowledge.

Leathard, A. *The Fight for Family Planning*. London, The Macmillan Press Ltd. 1980.

Masters, W. H. and Johnson, V. E. *Human Sexual Response*. London, J. and A. Churchill 1966.

Maude, Aylmer. *The Authorised Life of Marie C. Stopes*. London, Williams and Norgate 1924

McFarlane, K. B. *John Wycliffe and the Beginnings of English Non-Conformity*. London, English Universities Press 1952; Pelican Books 1972.

Norman, E. R. *Church and Society in England 1770-1970*. Oxford, Clarendon Press 1976.

Peel, J. and Potts, M. *Textbook of Contraceptive Practice*. Cambridge University Press 1967.

Rama Rau, D. *An Inheritance: The Memoirs of Dhanvanthi Rama Rau*. New York, Harper and Row; San Francisco, Hagerstown 1977. London, Heinemann 1978.

Sanger, M. *My Fight for Birth Control*. New York, Farrar Strauss 1932.

Sanger, M. *Margaret Sanger: An Autobiography*. London, Victor Gollancz 1939; New York, Dover 1971.

Stopes, M. *Married Love*. London, A. C. Fifield 1918.

Stopes, M. *Wise Parenthood*. London, A. C. Fifield 1918.

Stopes, M. *Radiant Motherhood*. London, G. P. Putnam's Sons 1920.

Stopes, M. *Enduring Passion*. London, G. P. Putnam's Sons 1928.

Suitters, B. *Be Brave and Angry. Chronicles of the International Planned Parenthood Federation*. International Planned Parenthood Federation. Printed Hertford: Stephen Austin and Sons 1973.

Spring Rice, M. *Working-Class Wives: Their Health and Conditions*. London, Penguin Books 1939; Virago Reprint Library No. 8 1981.

Sutherland, H. *Birth Control: A Statement of Christian Doctrine Against the Neo-Malthusians*. London, Harding and More 1922.

Van de Velde, Th. *Ideal Marriage: Its Physiology and Technique*. New York, Random House 1926; London, William Heinemann Medical Books 1930; Granada Publishing Ltd., in Mayflower Books 1972.

Wright, H. *The Sex Factor in Marriage*. London, Williams and Norgate Ltd. 1930.

Wright, H. *What is Sex? An Outline for Young People*. London, Williams and Norgate Ltd. 1935.

Wright, H. *Birth Control. Advice on Family Spacing and Healthy Sex Life*. London, Cassell & Co. 1935.

Wright, H. *More About the Sex Factor in Marriage* (later called *Sex Fulfilment in Married Women*) London, Williams and Norgate Ltd. 1947.

Wright, H. with the assistance of Wright H. B. *Contraceptive Technique. A Handbook for Medical Practitioners and Senior Students.* London, J & A Churchill Ltd. 1951.

Wright, H. *Sex and Society. A New Code of Sexual Behaviour.* London, George Allen and Unwin 1968.

Index

Note: numbers in italics refer to illustrations on pages facing numbers indicated.